The Forgotten Art of Healing
and Other Essays

To
Vera, for her love and care,
And for the happiness we share.

The Forgotten Art of Healing
and Other Essays

FAROKH ERACH UDWADIA
MD, FRCP (Edinburgh and London),
Master FCCP, FAMS, FACP, Hon. DSc

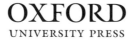

OXFORD
UNIVERSITY PRESS

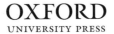

OXFORD

UNIVERSITY PRESS

YMCA Library Building, Jai Singh Road, New Delhi 110 001

Oxford University Press is a department of the University of Oxford. It furthers the
University's objective of excellence in research, scholarship, and education
by publishing worldwide in

Oxford New York

Auckland Cape Town Dar es Salaam Hong Kong Karachi Kuala Lumpur
Madrid Melbourne Mexico City Nairobi New Delhi Shanghai Taipei Toronto

With offices in
Argentina Austria Brazil Chile Czech Republic France Greece Guatemala
Hungary Italy Japan Poland Portugal Singapore South Korea Switzerland
Thailand Turkey Ukraine Vietnam

Oxford is a registered trademark of Oxford University Press
in the UK and in certain other countries

Published in India
by Oxford University Press, New Delhi

ISBN-13: 978-019-806174-8
ISBN-10: 019-806174-9

Typeset in Sabon LT Std 11/15
by Sai Graphic Design, New Delhi 110 055
Printed in India at EIH Limited, Haryana
Published by Oxford University Press
YMCA Library Building, Jai Singh Road, New Delhi 110 001

Contents

Preface

This book was written at the request of friends and colleagues who were keen that I express my views on medicine divorced from its medical and technical aspects. Yet, if one takes away science and technology from medicine is there anything left? Confronted by the hubris of great scientific achievements in medicine and in a world of changing values, many feel that medicine without its science and technology amounts to nothing or next to nothing. This is not true. There is an art to medicine, an art based on human values, which immeasurably enriches its science, an art which when combined with science not just cures, but also heals. Sadly, it has become an increasingly forgotten art and I felt an urge to express my views on it—hence the title of this book as also that of the first of the nine essays.

The advantages and disadvantages of contemporary medicine form a frequent topic of discussion among both the medical profession and the lay public. It is difficult to give a focused view on contemporary medicine, because one lives in the midst of its turmoil. Yet I was keen to dwell on three aspects of this subject. First, my reasons why in spite of the great advances in contemporary medicine, the medical profession is often looked upon with a certain degree of distrust and antagonism. Secondly, to stress the limits of medicine now and in the foreseeable future and finally to point out as Ivan Illich did several years ago, the increasing dependence of society on medicine and medical institutions, a dependence lucrative to the medical profession but of disadvantage to society.

If I write on Contemporary Medicine, I also need to discuss Medicine in the Future. There are many who believe with me that the future is now and that the seeds of the future have already been sown. This is with particular reference to genetic medicine. Will genetic science benefit man and medicine? Also, will the science of genetics tempt man to manipulate the human genome and set him hurtling along a new dangerous evolutionary path that changes Homo sapiens into a different unrecognizable species? There are no definite answers to these and many other questions.

An important topic related to medicine is Euthanasia and I have thought it fit to discuss various aspects of this question. Much can be said on both sides—for and against, but I hold the view with many others that reverence for life is a principle that should not be contravened.

Medical discoveries have always been a fascinating topic, particularly for the lay public. I have therefore written on Landmarks in Modern Medicine and on the Story of Anaesthesia. The former essay deals with the discovery of penicillin, of cortisone and of the structure of the DNA molecule. Keen observation, single-minded devotion and a spirit of inquiry lie at the heart of these discoveries. Yet there is an element of fortuitousness, an element of chance which made each of these discoveries possible.

Medicine has been influenced most of all by the natural sciences and also by many other human endeavours—notably philosophy, economics, art and religion. Perhaps my fascination and love for art prompted me to explore the relation between art and medicine, particularly the relationship between disease and artistic creativity. I have discussed this relationship with examples from Western art. Much as I wanted to, I sadly could not draw examples from Indian art, because the records on this subject are either meagre or nonexistent. I found this essay challenging and immensely satisfying and have thought it apt to illustrate it with pictures relating to Art and Medicine.

I have also written on Religion and Medicine, for religion has influenced medicine ever since it came into existence. Also, religion implies faith, and faith is an important cornerstone of medicine.

Finally, I have included in these nine essays my convocation address to the University of Benaras—the oldest existing university in the world. I do so because many students wished to see this address in print. I however do so with hesitation; because I would not like this address to be looked upon as a sermon. Yet I feel that I am old enough to offer words of advice to students on the threshold of their medical careers, if only to uphold values that lie at the heart of medicine.

I have read and consulted a number of books and references while writing these essays. They are too numerous to mention singly, but I would like to especially acknowledge P. Sandblom's book, *Creativity and Disease*, Bernard Lowne's book, *Lost Art of Healing*, James Le Fanu's book, *The Rise and Fall of Modern Medicine* and the issue on Death, Dying and the Medical duty (editors – G.R. Dinstan and P.J. Lachmann) in the British Medical Bulletin (Volume 52, April 1990). I have also made use of my own book, *Man and Medicine— A History*.

I owe a debt of gratitude to my wife, Vera for her patience and forbearance during the preparation of this work and for her reading and correcting the manuscript several times over. My very sincere thanks to Dr Khyati Mehta, my research assistant who has been associated with this work from its very inception. Her diligence and devotion were largely responsible for the completion of this book. I must also express my gratitude to my dear friend and distinguished surgeon , Dr Hirji S. Adenwalla. He has not only read the manuscript but offered excellent suggestions, many of which I have incorporated.

My thanks to Mr Neeraj Chavan for helping in the typing of the manuscript. I wish to acknowledge and thank the Wellcome Trust for the permission to print the pictures that illustrate the essay Art and Medicine. I also thank the Picasso Administration, Paris, who kindly agreed to grant permission for Picasso's canvas 'Science and Charity' to be used both as a cover for the book and as a plate section in the text. Finally, I thank Oxford University Press for their unstinted help and cooperation in publishing this work.

The Forgotten Art of Healing

May I never forget that the patient is a fellow creature in pain. May I never consider him merely a vessel of disease.

—MAIMONIDES

The stupendous advances of science and technology have changed the face of medicine. Medicine is capable of performing amazing feats deemed incredible 50 years ago. Yet paradoxically there is today a deepening disillusion, distrust and even antagonism against medicine and the medical profession. The paradox is indeed striking for around the middle of the last century when science and technology hovered merely in the background and medicine had achieved little, the profession was held in the highest regard and the doctor's image outshone that of any other profession. Today, when science and technology envelop medicine in an all-embracing grasp and when medicine has achieved a great deal, the respect for the profession has plummeted and the image of the physician is increasingly tarnished. To my mind the main reason for this paradox is because medicine has strayed from its path, has lost its way, has lost its goal. The mechanization of medicine, the hubris of its technology and science has submerged its art, robbed it of its raison d'etre, its humanism.

The physician no longer ministers to a distinctive person, but concerns himself with separate malfunctioning organs. The distressed patient, the human being, is frequently forgotten or relegated to the background.

In these days of burgeoning science, the medical student and the doctor are both absorbed in the intricacies of technological advances related to medicine. Yet medicine is learnt and taught at the bedside by listening and talking to the patients, by touching and examining them; not just from books, not from gleaming machines and sophisticated gadgetry, nor from the rapturous attention to beautiful images obtained through computerized or magnetic resonance imaging (MRI), endoscopies, angiographies or from other wonderful gifts of science and technology. Both science and technology are essential features of modern medicine, forces that have given medicine a quantum leap into the twenty-first century. But there is more to medicine than its science and its technology. Technology cannot substitute for a carefully taken history or a meticulously performed physical examination. Technology will not help cement a doctor-patient relationship, nor will it assuage the mental torment, fear, anxiety that may follow in the wake of an illness.

This brief essay is an attempt to express the essence of the art behind medicine. It is difficult to do so. For one, the art is intrinsically mixed with its science, for another the art behind medicine has no physical attributes (so easy to detect and describe) but abstract qualities of the mind and heart which blend to vibrate in empathy with an ill individual contributing significantly to healing. Finally, it is an art which today has been pushed aside by the triumphs of modern science. It is lurking now in the shadows, a forgotten art, perhaps in time to come, (it may well be) a lost art. But it is nevertheless an essential art that needs to be resurrected and shown the light of day.

A little over 25 centuries ago, Hippocrates proclaimed, 'For where there is the love of man, there is also the love of art. For some patients, though conscious that their position is perilous, recover their health, simply through their contentment with the physician'. How very true this is even today—one has only to ask a patient who loves and trusts his doctor to discover the truth of this counsel. Paracelsus, the renowned Renaissance physician who lived and worked in the sixteenth century included among the basic requisites of a physician, 'intuition which is necessary to understand the patient, his body, his disease. He must have the feel and touch which make it possible for him to be in sympathetic communication with the patient's spirit'. This last sentence epitomizes the intangible qualities that lie at the heart of medicine.

How does a doctor even begin to achieve this 'sympathetic communication with a patient's spirit?' It is first and foremost by listening to the patient who seeks help—taking a good history. Taking a patient's history is a forgotten art; yet a good history very often gives the diagnosis or hides the clue to the solution of a very difficult problem. The art of history-taking can never be perfectly mastered, even by the most accomplished physician. A disease often does not run true to type, in that the same disease may manifest differently in different patients. Each patient is a unique individual; his response to disease may well be unique. This response depends not just on the disease process but on the physiological alterations and the adaptation to physiological change; it is conditioned by the genetic make-up, the environment, constitution, physical endurance, emotional and mental state and perhaps by several other unknown protean factors. Also, each patient interprets what happens to him or her in a unique way and the expression in words to the doctor of what he or she feels may take different forms. For the doctor to be able to distinguish the relevant from the irrelevant, to separate the chaff from the grain, so as to touch the heart of the matter is indeed a challenging task. If he succeeds in doing so he often makes the correct diagnosis or is at least aware in which direction to proceed. A poor history, whatever be the reason, is a great handicap. It leaves the doctor puzzled, sailing on uncharted seas, not knowing where to turn.

I have often been asked by many students—'what is the secret of a good history?'. First and foremost, it is listening to the patient, hearing him patiently, encouraging him to speak. The art of listening is therefore an art within an art. To listen effectively one must listen not just with ears, but with one's whole self, with all of one's senses, for then only will a trained physician hear an unspoken problem. It is not enough to ferret the nature of a patient's disease; it is equally important while listening, to assess his emotional state, to get to know the province of his mind which could either colour his disease or actually be responsible for his complaints. Listening can provide a therapeutic catharsis for a patient, an education for the doctor and is thus often the secret of healing.

The importance of listening to a patient's family history, social, personal and marital history cannot be overstressed. A good listener will gently be able to make his patient speak about his hopes, ambitions, successes, his frustrations and failures. Only then will the doctor engage with the patient holistically, as a human being, rather than merely concentrate on the dysfunction of various organ systems.

After listening comes questioning—also an art in itself. Questions need to be carefully worded. There are some patients who would agree with all a physician asks—they love to please the doctor. There are some who overplay one or more symptoms, only to deceive the doctor; there are others who are taciturn and who need to be coaxed gently, cleverly to open up. They often underplay their symptoms and sometimes unwittingly hide the life-threatening seriousness of an underlying problem. And then there are some who mask their problems in a mass of irrelevant disconnected verbiage. A clue to their problems may lie buried within a plethora of words, or in a sentence muttered as an aside. There the physician needs to apply the brake, ask precise questions and await precise answers. Perhaps the greatest difficulty with patients is that so many are anxious, tense and nervous, partly from fear that they harbour a dreadful disease, fear of the physician, and what the physician will do to them. The art of the physician is to know how to put them at ease before starting with the history.

It is often forgotten that all patients respond to genuine kindness, they all hope to find a genuine, sympathetic friend in their physician. Only then will they give the physician their full confidence. And then there comes, little by little or sometimes in torrents, a story often disjointed, but which when pieced together throws light on the innermost recesses of a human life, and perhaps also discloses the reason for a problematic illness.

The art of medicine is in assessing the patient as a whole—the mind and the body. Many patients come with complaints referred to an organ-system, but whose true origin is due to a disturbance in the mind—the result of stress, worry, conflicts and frustrations, that often plague modern existence. To fail to recognize this is to perpetuate the patient's problem, to order expensive tests that could be ruinous to a poor family and to induce the patient to shop from doctor to doctor. Let me illustrate this with a recent example.

Miss A, a 23-year-old lady working in a software company was brought by her lady employer to see me for recurrent abdominal pain, weight loss and an oral temperature of 99°F starting two years ago. She had seen many doctors, had all tests done—these included blood tests, stool tests, endoscopies, ultrasound examination of the abdomen, computerized tomography (CT) imaging of the chest and the abdomen. She had been given numerous drugs and the gastroenterologist had finally made a tentative diagnosis of TB of the abdomen and had started her off on anti-TB treatment. She awaited a laparoscopy of the abdomen and was brought to me for advice. A good history was difficult; she was withdrawn, taciturn and answered in monosyllables. I found no clue from the way she described her abdominal pain. I decided to concentrate on features outside her complaints. To start with, I complimented her on having graduated under difficult conditions; she had graduated and done higher studies through a correspondence course and had secured a job which paid her handsomely. I talked of her school, the kind of studies she opted for, her activities during the day as she grew up. She then as an aside admitted to having very little sleep. She would fall asleep at 4 am and had to get up at 6 am to prepare to go to work. 'Why should a girl as young as you, working the whole day not fall fast asleep at night?' I asked her. The question was greeted by silence. She admitted to no worry, no anxieties and said she was happy. I then talked of her ambitions, her desires and what she planned to do as the years went on. For the first time she spoke a little animatedly about her job and an expected promotion with a further increase in her salary. 'But is that all a young girl wants in life? Don't you want to get married, have a home, have lovely children?' I had touched a tender chord. A silent tear rolled down her cheek, and she bit her lip so as not to cry. 'This is not likely to happen,' she said in a whisper. 'Please tell me why—if you do, I promise to get you well.' Then it came out in a rush. Her father, an untrained electrician earned next to nothing. He was unemployed, worked part time when some temporary work was available. Her mother was uneducated but kept the family together. She had two younger sisters and one younger brother, all in school. They all lived in a small single room. Her salary, however, sufficed to run the house, educate (at a good school) her brother and sisters. The whole family was hopelessly dependent on her. To marry and start a family of her own would plunge her parents into abject poverty. She could never bring herself to do this. The conflict in her mind now surfaced—she talked, I listened, and then explained gently that this was a natural conflict, a personal dilemma and it was responsible for both her abdominal complaints and insomnia. When a patient recognizes the root cause of a problem, it becomes the first step to the solution of the problem, and if the problem is unsolvable, it helps the patient to come to terms with it.

There was now a sweet smile on her face, a smile of gratitude perhaps for someone who had listened to her story. I examined her and found no abnormality on clinical examination, nor in the extensive expensive tests that had been repeatedly performed on her. Seated once again in front of me, I asked if she saw any solution to her problem. 'No!' was the monosyllabic answer. I next looked at the lady employer who I noticed was quite moved by the story. I realized that she must be a kind woman to have taken the trouble to arrange for the young girl to see me and to accompany her for the consultation. I then spoke to her, 'You are the only one who can change this girl's fortune as also that of the family. You must be kind to have brought this girl to me. You will have earned the gratitude of many, mine included and earned the blessings of the Lord if you can employ on a decent salary the father of this young lady in your factory.' He is an untrained electrician but he is young, could be trained and be profitably employed. Will you not please do this for all of us?' The lady nodded her head in assent and embraced her employee. It had been a dreadful day for me to start with—a cardiac arrest in the ICU and very ill patients deciding to get more ill as the day went on. The day ended on a happy note—I felt uplifted and could not stop smiling.

Let me give just one more example how 'listening' to the patient can be of great help. A middle-aged man consulted me for purpura of undetermined origin. Purpura is a disease characterized by bleeding under the skin, from mucous membranes and rarely within organ systems. Investigations had revealed that his purpura was due to a fall in his platelet count to 30,000/mm^3, the normal count being 150,000-300,000/ mm^3. He had seen several haematologists to determine the cause of his purpura. All blood and other tests, including a bone marrow examination were non-contributory to the cause. He was therefore diagnosed as idiopathic thrombocytopenic purpura. In lay terms this means purpura due to a fall in the platelet count, the cause of which is undetermined (idiopathic). He was to begin treatment for this and consulted me before doing so.

I took a relevant history of his complaints and then came to his personal and social history. 'Do you smoke Mr B ?' 'Yes, about 10 cigarettes a day,' he replied. 'Do you drink?' I asked him. 'Yes, I do,' he replied. Perhaps absent-mindedly, I questioned, 'What do you drink?' 'I used to drink three pegs of whiskey daily but I have now switched to gin and tonic.' 'Why have you changed from whiskey to gin?' I asked. 'I was told that my alcohol consumption would hurt me, so I changed to gin and tonic which I feel has less spirit than whiskey,' he answered with a smile. 'I am not quite sure Mr B whether your assumption is correct.' Mr B then warmed up to the subject of gin and tonic. He said that he now loved his gin and indeed had also grown very fond of the tonic. He would drink tonic water during the day very often even without the gin. His wife now joined the conversation and said that her husband had been drinking more than four bottles of 'tonic' daily for the last several months. 'More tonic and hardly any water,' was her comment.

A bell started to ring furiously in my mind. Had we stumbled on something unusual? One of the common causes of a low platelet count is exposure to drugs which in some patients produce antibodies which destroy platelets—a form of a hypersensitivity reaction. Even exposure to a very small quantity of the offending drug could then result in a lowered platelet count and purpura. 'Tonic' contains very small amounts of quinine, and quinine is one drug commonly known to cause a lowered platelet count (thrombocytopenia) through an allergic or hypersensitivity reaction.

I then examined Mr B and found nothing other than many purpuric (bleeding) spots under the skin. With a broad smile on my face, I sat him again in front of me and said, 'I just want you to do one thing for me, Mr B. Stop your 'tonic' completely and consume your gin with 'lime' or any other soft drink. Do this for three weeks, repeat the platelet count and then come and see me.' 'Mrs B, please ensure that your husband follows my instructions.'

Three weeks later Mr and Mrs B came and saw me again. They were smiling happily. The purpuric spots had disappeared and the platelet count had risen to normal levels. 'This is indeed miraculous!' said Mrs B. 'Not so,' I replied. I explained how quinine in the tonic could have been responsible for his problem. 'There is one way we can prove this for sure, provided your husband agrees to take a small risk. We shall challenge him with a small dose of quinine taken orally and if his platelets fall again and purpura reappears, we shall know for sure that the quinine in the tonic that he used to drink was responsible for the problem.' Mr B accepted the challenge, took the small dose of quinine orally and within three days broke out with a purpuric rash with a sharp fall in his platelets. It took three to four weeks for the platelets to return to normal levels and his purpuric rash to disappear. I had never come across a patient such as this and I doubt if I ever will. Listening and questioning and listening again provided the vital clue; no gadgetry, machine or other tests could have possibly unearthed the cause of Mr B's problem.

The complexities in the art behind a good patient history are further illustrated by the fact that the chief complaint a patient comes with does not necessarily point to or reflect the seat of disease. The chief complaint may be abdominal pain, yet the seat of the disease could be in the chest, or could be related to a metabolic or an endocrine disorder. Pain in the shoulder may be due to the heart and yet chest pain could be related to anxiety, stress and mental conflict rather than to the heart. In this age of triumphant science, patients to start with often seek aid from a specialist. A specialist is of immense help, but his field is narrow and the more specialized he is, the narrower becomes his field of expertise. Disease, however, is no specialist. A patient does not come to a physician pointing to his liver, spleen or kidney and even if he does so, he is often wrong. He comes because he feels ill, and in the early stage of an illness , his symptoms are often vague and unless viewed in a holistic perspective, may be misleading. It is therefore to the patient's advantage in the first place to seek aid from one whose daily practice covers the whole gamut of medicine. A holistic view of the patient and his disease is vital—it combines both the art and science of medicine. A specialist enters when the problem behind an illness has been clearly defined and needs either specialized tests or specialized management.

The Basis of Clinical Diagnosis

The cornerstones of a good clinical diagnosis are a good history, a thorough clinical examination and relevant investigations interpreted in the light of knowledge and experience. Diagnostic talent has to be assiduously cultivated. Method, the acquisition of factual knowledge, keen observation and an intelligent assimilation of past experience at the bedside are some of its absolute prerequisites. Today, the lost art of history-taking is associated with a similar lacuna in the ability to elicit physical findings. This is because there is a lack of emphasis on the importance of a good, complete, physical examination. Perhaps the curriculum in the universities is heavily loaded towards teaching the scientific advances of modern medicine, leaving very little time for bedside clinical medicine. Students and even graduates of medicine often do not know how to palpate an enlarged spleen, or elicit the ankle jerk in a correct manner, or distinguish bronchial from vesicular breathing, or recognize the blowing diastolic murmur of aortic incompetence or recognize a distended enlarged gall bladder— just to cite a few examples. Yet they may perhaps correctly interpret pressure readings of a catheter study of the right or left heart, or know what to expect in the electromyography (EMG) of a patient with motor neurone disease.

A good clinical examination is both an art and a science. The art lies in eliciting physical findings; the science rests in their proper interpretation. Knowledge of the significance of physical signs alone is valueless unless it is combined with the art and expertise that detect these signs. A physician should therefore cultivate his sense of sight; his ability to hear, feel and smell; his ability to process what he has sensed in his brain, his ability to recall his past experiences with reference to the present situation, to weigh, to judge and to then arrive at the root cause of a patient's dangerous illness. The good clinician uses these abilities methodically, efficiently, and through intelligent practice almost unconsciously. He can only do so if he is trained in the art and science of a good clinical examination. In the words of Osler, 'Learn to see, learn to hear, learn to feel, learn to smell and know that by practice alone you can become perfect. Medicine is learnt at the bedside and not in the classroom. Let not your conception of the manifestation of disease come from words heard in the lecture room or read in a book. See and then reason and compare and control. But see first.'

No clinical observation however small or trivial should be considered as unimportant. It should not be set aside just because it does not fit with a clinical diagnosis. It needs to be explained. A physician solving a difficult clinical problem is akin to a detective unravelling a difficult crime. As the famous detective Hercule Poirot in Agatha Christie's novel, *The Mysterious Affair at Styles* said, 'Beware! Peril to the detective who says, "It is too small – it does not matter. It will not agree. I will forget it." That way lies confusion – everything matters!'

Let me briefly illustrate the art of physical examination and its importance in clinical diagnosis by two case studies.

A young officer in the merchant navy was transferred from Sri Lanka to our unit for psychiatric care. While on his ship he showed psychotic behaviour. He was rowdy, querulous, talked irrelevantly and continuously. He was at times manic in his speech and behaviour and at times depressed, morose, silent. He exhibited strong suicidal tendencies and had to be physically restrained. A clinical examination and all relevant tests including imaging studies done at Sri Lanka showed no cause for his behaviour. He was transferred with a diagnosis of manic depressive psychosis and was advised electroconvulsive therapy. A detailed history was unfortunately unavailable. There were just three physical findings on a careful physical examination. An axillary temperature of 99.5° F, a faint but definite butterfly rash on the face and a mucosal ulcer at the junction of the hard and soft palate. These findings suggested a possibility of systemic lupus erythromatosis, an uncommon disease, rare in males, that could cause psychotic behaviour. Relevant investigations directed towards the diagnosis, confirmed the presence of the disease. He was appropriately treated and made an excellent recovery. A thorough scientific knowledge of this uncommon disease would have proved of no avail if the few relevant signs had not been detected.

The second example is of a middle-aged man who presented with a life-threatening emergency. He was admitted in another hospital to start with for severe pain in the chest and the middle of the back. He was diagnosed as an acute myocardial infarct. On the second day of his admission he was reported to have suffered a cardiac arrest from which he was resuscitated with difficulty. After resuscitation, an X-ray of his chest showed a fairly large pleural effusion (fluid within the pleural space) which on tapping revealed heavily blood-stained fluid. A drain was inserted into the pleural space and the patient was transferred to our unit at Breach Candy Hospital. He had been transfused with blood to counter a sharp fall in his haemoglobin before his transfer. The pleural effusion had been put down to pulmonary embolism (a clot travelling from either the heart or the leg veins and obstructing a vessel within the lung). There were just two physical findings that gave a clue to the correct diagnosis. The first was very poor arterial pulsations in both lower limbs and the other was a 'bruit' or 'murmur' heard with the stethoscope over the middle of the back to the left of the midline. This pointed to a dissection of the aorta (a tear in the wall of the aorta—the large vessel arising from the heart). A 'catheter study' was ordered to prove the diagnosis.

The catheter study was reported to be normal. But the two clinical signs together with the history were too obvious to be ignored. We therefore asked for a CT chest which proved the diagnosis. The CT chest showed a tear in the aortic wall and a dissection of the wall starting just below the aortic arch and extending right down beyond the bifurcation of the aorta, thereby obstructing blood flow to both the lower limbs. The cardiac arrest and the collection of large bloody pleural fluid before he was transferred to our hospital was due to a partial rupture of the dissected aorta into the pleural space. It was the sudden loss of blood which in fact had produced a marked fall in the blood pressure and a cardiac arrest. The importance of the art of eliciting physical findings led to a correct diagnosis, appropriate management with ultimate recovery.

The process of making a diagnosis starts at the first contact with the patient. It crystallizes by the time the history is over. The history points the way, the physical examination then confirms it, or occasionally points to another path. It is bad medicine to fit jigsaw pieces together, treating the history as one entity, the physical findings as another and the investigations when performed still another. The logical process beginning with the history should be smooth and structured so that by the time a physician finishes examining the patient, the probable diagnosis has been made. Therein lies the art of medicine.

Some lucky physicians are blessed with an extra-sharp clinical sense, a true 'clinical instinct'. 'Clinical instinct' involves the ability to arrive at a definite conclusion without a conscious logical process. It perhaps depends on buried past experiences without conscious remembrance, so that the physician relates a clinical problem that he encounters in the present to a pattern he has already experienced one or more times in the past without conscious effort.

Relevant Investigations

Investigations are often necessary to substantiate a clinical diagnosis or to help differentiate one possible diagnosis from another or to aid in the management of a clinical problem. Investigations should never take the place of a good clinical history and a thorough physical examination. To start with, they should be simple and should always remain essential and relevant to the problem being investigated. Clinical judgement and not routine procedures should dictate the nature of investigations.

Investigations come under the realm of science and often involve the use of sophisticated gadgetry and machines. At times the latter are of invaluable benefit and show what human faculties cannot detect. A good clinician must, however, be perfectly acquainted with sources of error that can creep into the results of sophisticated tests. If the result of an investigation does not fit a clinical diagnosis based on sound reason and logic, the wise physician repeats the investigation rather than change his diagnosis. This is not to denigrate the value of essential investigations. It is merely to look at their value in the correct perspective. There is no doubt that science and technology which drive modern medicine, have led to the over-investigation of patients, often through invasive procedures, using complex machines. The cost-benefit ratio of many such investigations performed all over the world is indeed poor. Over-investigation to my mind is a form of mental bankruptcy. It dehumanizes medicine, threatens to reduce it to the level of a machine-patient relationship and effectively negates the art behind medicine.

CLINICAL JUDGEMENT

A physician must needs be a judge. Judgement is difficult, for indeed medicine has been defined as the 'art of coming to a conclusion on insufficient evidence'. It is no surprise that errors in judgement frequently abound. Clinical judgement does not come either within the purview of art or science. It is a special quality, a faculty—often inborn and occasionally cultivated. It cannot be equated to intellectual ability for it may be lacking in brilliant minds and be present to a marked degree in those who in other respects are far less clever or knowledgeable. Sir Robert Hutchinson regards it 'much the same as common sense and closely allied to a sense of humour, which is the same thing as a sense of proportion. Those who lack it are apt to fail to see the wood from the trees'.

To cope with the diagnosis and management of an illness, in particular a life-threatening emergency, requires more than mere factual knowledge, reason, logic, experience and skill. It requires good clinical judgement—the hallmark of a good physician. Clinical judgement is a rich blend of all the above requisites and adds to these a further, intangible, indefinable quality; a quality that encompasses faith, charity, hope and compassion; a quality that has a deep understanding of human nature; a quality that can reach out to and sustain the shattered morale or the broken spirit of a seriously ill human being. It is also the quality that gives the doctor in crisis, the wisdom to know what to say and do and what not to say and do; when to wait and watch, and when to treat vigorously without delay; when to fight death and when to give in to it; when to press for cure and when to console with words or to rest content with palliative relief. Sound clinical judgement includes an extra-special perceptive ability that enables a doctor to 'sense' a clue which his less fortunate colleagues will miss; the ability to process this clue and judge its correct diagnostic, therapeutic and prognostic implications. Such a clue need not be abstruse or esoteric. It is generally simple, but simple only to those who have eyes to see. It may be obvious in the anguish on the patient's brow, or the despair and defeat in his eyes or in the rattle in his chest and throat. It may be evident in the detection of a few purpuric spots, in the change in the character of the pulse or the breathing, or in the size of a pupil. It may lie in the failure to relieve an important symptom, or persistence of an ominous sign, or in the detection of new symptoms and signs. A physician who combines the sharpness of his perceptive faculties with a wisdom born of reading and experience, with a compassion for and an understanding of human suffering and who also possesses the faculty of good clinical judgement is truly blessed by the gods. He has an attribute which no machine can duplicate and no science can invent. A physician with these attributes (by physician I include a doctor in any field) enjoys a ringside seat in the theatre of life. The world is a stage and he has the most intimate insight into many who cross this stage and seek his help. He also has the ability and the wisdom to alter for the better the drama of their lives. Physicians today seek honours and rewards. These may be welcome when deserved and due. But what greater honour and reward is there than to help release the grip of death and strengthen the hold on life in an ill individual entrusted to his care? What greater joy and satisfaction than to see the smile of relief and gratitude in those near and dear to such an individual! I do believe that to be a physician under such circumstances is an unmatched privilege.

Patient Care

'Care' implies much more than the use of medications, procedures, surgical interventions or other marvels of science in patient management. 'Care' can only come if the physician has an empathy for his patient. Empathy is not just sympathy; it implies a 'feeling' of deep concern for the overall welfare of the patient prompting help in every conceivable way so as to restore the patient's health or mitigate suffering. Empathy on the part of the physician is recognized intuitively by the patient, who reciprocates with faith and trust, forging thereby a two-way relationship, the proverbial bond between doctor and patient. Faith and trust cannot be quantified or tested; they are abstract attributes of the mind, but they unquestionably help in healing. This has been the experience of physicians from Hippocratic times, right down to the present scientific age. How does faith act? I do not know the science of its action but perhaps it influences the mind to act on the body helping it to heal through neuroendocrine pathways. The mind-body relationship is comparatively speaking an unexplored field. Future science may perhaps explain and unravel this relationship.

A caring physician is often rewarded with success. It is remarkable how a critically ill conscious individual who hovers between life and death has antennae which recognizes and latches on to the empathy shown by a physician who truly cares. It is also amazing how such a patient can distinguish true concern from mere outward sympathy.

Concern and care shown by the treating physician are supports that boost morale, instil hope and confidence, enabling the patient to fight death and perchance survive.

Good patient care necessitates that the patient actively participates in his own management. For that he needs to be well informed, his rights respected, options in management clearly discussed, and the possible untoward effects of drugs and interventional procedures carefully explained. Active patient participation is the key to the successful resolution of difficult problems. Yet the wise physician knows what to tell and what not to tell. The attitude of the physician in this regard depends to an extent on the social mores, culture, traditions, expectations of the society in which he practises.

THE FORGOTTEN ART

Today, science rules; however, the practice of its science without an equal measure of its art dehumanizes medicine, robs it of its essence. This is unfortunately the trend today which needs must be reversed. The art of medicine lies in the application of its science to the overall holistic care of an individual patient.

A physician steeped in the art knows the value of kindness, sympathy and caring in the healing of a patient. The art of medicine remains all-pervasive even when its science fails or has reached its utmost limits. For when all the marvels of science are of no avail to unfortunately ward off the fatal end, 'it is no small portion of a physician's art to rid his patient's path of thorns if he cannot make it bloom with roses.'

The art of medicine lies in hearing an unspoken subtle nuance in a patient's history and in the ability to spot and appreciate the significance of one or more subtle physical signs that no gadget or machine could possibly recognize. It also lies in the ability of a physician to sift the evidence before him and give the right answer (of several possible answers) to the appropriate question. The art of medicine (even though the scientist might scoff at him) also lies in the intuitive feel for a solution either in diagnosis or management. Above all it consists of looking at a sick patient holistically and in assessing not just the body but also the mind. The art of medicine is the art of healing, not just treating, not even just curing. *Yet it is only when art and science join hands that healing is best accomplished. It is only then that a physician can engage the unique individuality of a particular human being so that a sick patient becomes much more than an illness or a disease that needs to be treated.* A broader engagement between the doctor and the patient gives a holistic perspective, lends clarity to judgement and helps overcome the difficulties of decision-making. It bonds the doctor and the patient in a mutual trusting relationship, reinforcing an unwritten covenant hallowed by time.

Let me end my plea for reviving the forgotten art of healing by echoing a statement made by Trousseau, a famous French physician, in an era where in fact there was very little science. He ended one of his lectures in clinical medicine thus—

'For mercy's sake gentlemen, let us have a little less science and a little more art'.

Convocation Address at the
Benaras Hindu University (2004)

Prof. P. Ramachandra Rao, Vice-Chancellor of the Benaras Hindu University, Dr. Mohanty, Director, Institute of Medical Sciences, Faculty Members, Colleagues, Students, Ladies and Gentlemen,

I would like to thank you for the honour you have conferred upon me by awarding me the Doctorate of Science of this prestigious university and by requesting me to deliver the convocation address at today's function. I see eager young faces before me; young men and women hopefully equipped by this august university to embark and sail the uncharted sea of life. I feel a sense of nostalgia; fond memories crowd on to me, for I remember the day I joined medical school many many years ago, when my fellow-students and I sat, as you sit now, and listened with rapt attention to the valedictory address of a distinguished teacher.

Let me take you back to your roots. Ancient India exclusively practised Ayurvedic medicine. The three great centres of all learning were Taxila, Nalanda and Benaras. Taxila, founded in the sixth century BC, was reportedly the most famous, and some of the greatest men in ancient India graduated from Taxila or were teachers of this university. They include Chanakya, Panini, Jivaka and Nagarajuna.

Nalanda was a university town which at its peak (between fifth to twelfth century AD) had 40,000 students and 1,500 teachers in a campus, a mile long and half a mile wide.

Benaras was as ancient and as famous as Taxila and Nalanda. However, while Taxila and Nalanda faded and disappeared as centres of learning with the passage of time, Benaras continued to flourish and is ranked today as the oldest surviving university in the whole world. Those who have studied and have passed out of this ancient university and those who teach are indeed the torchbearers of a great and ancient tradition. May this tradition be kept forever alive and may its values be cherished for all time.

I wish to address you today on two subjects. The first is to give you my thoughts on the attributes of a good physician, and the second is to give you a panoramic view of the changing face of medicine—the past, the present and the future.

Unquestionably, a physician (and by the word 'physician', I include a doctor practising any speciality he or she chooses), must needs be competent. It is the university and its teachers which provide and equip you with this competence. However, the acquisition of a degree in my opinion is merely a licence to practise medicine or your chosen speciality. Your consummation as a physician can only come after you have gone out into the world of sickness and suffering and grappled long with death and disease. Unless the unfortunate values of present-day living have poisoned your mind, dulled your sensibilities and blunted your sympathies, you will learn that there is more to a true physician than the mere knowledge of the science of medicine. It is only when the art and philosophy of medicine have encrusted science, and have permeated into its very core that you will have blossomed into a true physician. Bear in mind that competence needs to be perpetually reinforced and renewed. A physician is first and foremost a student for life. 'Young and old, we are all undergraduates in the school of experience.'

I will not detail what constitutes competence. But I would urge you in this machine-age not to forget the use of your eyes, ears and hands. None are so blind as those who have eyes and yet not see, or so deaf as those who have ears and yet not hear, or so unfeeling as those who have touch and yet not feel. The art and science of medicine is not taught by books; it is acquired only if you have lived with disease and made your home at the bedside of patients.

Competence, however, is not enough. Competence must be associated in even greater measure with what is best termed 'humanity'. Humanity is the sensibility which enables a physician to feel for the distress and suffering of a patient, prompting him to provide relief. Humanity embraces both care and compassion; it forms the core of a doctor-patient relationship, a relationship which has been increasingly eroded in our present age.

Honesty and integrity are other attributes integral to a physician. The need for honesty and integrity in all matters pertaining to patients and to the outside world is obvious enough. I however refer specially to intellectual honesty. Self-delusion comes easy to one and all in medicine and I too admit to the crime of Procrustes. Procrustes was a robber who had become an innkeeper. When a traveller stopped for the night at his inn, Procrustes would show him to his bed. When the guest was asleep the robber would determine how the guest fitted the bed. If he was short, he would bind him and stretch him so as to fit the bed; if he was too long he would chop off his legs so that he fitted the bed. In medicine it is common to jump to a preformed diagnosis and then delude yourself by making the clinical features fit this diagnosis. You add to what is not or subtract from what is, in order to justify a hasty preformed conclusion.

To err is human, and there is no physician on earth who has not made mistakes. The best-trained faculties may falter in observation, and even in the most experienced, errors in judgement must inevitably occur in an art and science which often consists in the balancing of probabilities. Cultivate an honesty of mind which recognizes, regrets and proclaims these mistakes. Only then will you learn from them and perhaps not repeat them. Do not hide your mistakes under a bushel or pretend that they never existed. If you do so, you will be increasingly unable to recognize truth; you will tread the unfortunate path of self-deception and delusion and your mistakes will multiply.

Can there be a true doctor who does not practise charity? Unquestionably not. Never refuse a patient who seeks your help but cannot afford your fees. You will be twice blessed—both by the patient and by the Lord who values the poor more than the rich. You have the right to live in reasonable comfort but let me quote you a pertinent saying—'No one should approach the temple of science with the soul of a money-changer'.

Then comes humility, the hallmark of a true physician. The grace of humility is a precious gift. 'Knowledge is proud that he knows so much, Wisdom is humble that he knows no more'. Extend your charity, humility and consideration not only to your patients, but also to your colleagues, so that you do unto them as you would have them do unto you.

In my opinion, what distinguishes a great physician from an ordinary one is the power of judgement. Hippocrates said 'Judgement is difficult, and indeed medicine has been defined as the art of coming to a conclusion on insufficient evidence'. We can increase our power of observation by constant practice. We can become more knowing and more wise through study and experience, but can we improve on our judgement? To an extent, judgement is an inborn faculty; 'the result of a union of mind and character, which a man either has or has not, and it is almost as difficult for him to increase it as to add a cubit to his stature'.

Perhaps the only way to help improve judgement is to improve our mind, not by scientific training alone, but by an exposure to art, culture, literature, history, philosophy—the other great fields of human endeavour. A broader study of the humanities will enable you to understand Man and his afflictions far better than the detailed study of medicine alone. Dip therefore into the treasures of the world around you. Medicine is the study of Man. Study mankind and you will have enhanced your study of Man.

Last but not the least we come to an important attribute of every good physician or surgeon—Equanimity or Aequanimitas, as Sir William Osler termed it. Equanimity means imperturbability, the ability to be unruffled, to be cool, calm amid stress and storm, to be clear in thinking and judgement, during an emergency, or during grave crisis or peril. It is the ability not to betray the emotions of worry, anxiety and above all of fear when treating critically ill patients. Some physicians are born with the gift of aequanimitas, some cultivate it with practice and experience. To be possessed of true equanimity within and without is a divine gift. But even if you cannot help the storm that rages within you, train yourself to hide this, so that you present a picture of fortitude and calm from which your patient imbibes sustenance and strength.

So there you have it, ladies and gentlemen. I give you Competence and Humanity, Honesty and Integrity, Charity, Humility, Judgement, Equanimity. Nurture these qualities as best as you can, so that they are part of you, inseparable from you and you will have followed in the great footsteps of Charaka and Susruta.

Let me now give you a kaleidoscopic picture of the changing face of medicine—its past and its present; permit me also to peer through the mists of uncertainty into the future. The past, present and future are intrinsically linked. Let me quote:

'Time present and time past
Are both perhaps present in time future
And time future contained in time past'.

Medicine is as old as man. The trail of medicine stretches back into the mists of time. It has witnessed several twists and turns, victories and defeats, periods of scintillating light and sombre darkness. After several millennia of recorded history, medicine has now evolved into a powerful force, an art, a science, and a profession that has made a quantum leap into the twenty-first century. The roots of medicine lie in magic—in the magical and religious beliefs of the shamans and priest physicians of the civilizations of antiquity. It was, however, philosophy which gave the first true impetus to the evolution of medicine. The Vedas in India and the great Greek philosophers in the West asked pertinent questions—Who is Man? Where does he come from, where does he go, how does he relate to nature and his environment? Religion and philosophy struck deep roots for medicine, but it was the advances in the natural sciences that nourished these roots, so that over several centuries medicine grew into a beautiful blend of art and science.

The panorama of medicine, its evolution through five millennia is not just a chronological sequence of events and discoveries. The romance of medicine lies in the dynamic cavalcade of men and women who walked its trail. It is embodied in the heroes and imposters, the caring and uncaring who shaped its path. The triumphs of modern medicine have been built brick by brick on the foundations laid by these past heroes of medicine. Our success today rests squarely on the shoulders of many of our great ancestors. We have indeed an ancestry to be truly proud of and we must acknowledge this with gratitude. I urge you to learn and get to know more about some of these great men who have shaped our path. If you do so you will be inspired by their devotion, compassion, wisdom, skill, perseverance and their spirit of inquiry. Let me just mention a few of these stalwarts crowned in the Valhalla of Medicine.

We start with Imhotep, the first great physician in recorded history—an Egyptian who lived around 2700 BC. He was truly a Renaissance man in the age of antiquity—a man who besides being a great and kind physician was also a scribe, a philosopher, and an architect. The people of Egypt lined the banks of the Nile and wept as his funeral barge went down the river. We then continue with Hippocrates, the Father of Medicine who founded clinical bedside medicine, emphasized the art of history-taking, of careful observation, use of the eyes, ears and hands, and who gave us the Hippocratic Oath. Then we come to our own Charaka and Susruta who were the pillars of medicine and surgery respectively in ancient India, embodying their work in their 'Samhitas.' Let me proceed further and remind you of some other great heroes of medicine—Andreas Vesalius, a rebel of the Renaissance period, who in his early twenties founded the science of anatomy; Ambroise Paré, another rebel in the same period, a barber surgeon, who among other discoveries devised the ligature to stop arterial bleeding from injuries and wounds; Jenner, a countryside practitioner who discovered vaccination against smallpox, a scourge the world is rid of today, but a scourge which decimated vast populations in the past; Hunter who further pioneered surgery; Lister who discovered antisepsis and asepsis; Semmelweis, a man ignored and even scorned during his life who showed that mere hand-washing sharply reduced the incidence and mortality of puerperal sepsis. Closer to our era we have William Osler, a complete physician who combined within himself the qualities of knowledge, wisdom, the spirit of inquiry and compassion. I would also urge you to remember that great contributions to medicine have been made by scientists not within the fold of the medical profession. Perhaps the greatest of these scientists was Louis Pasteur, a French chemist, who theorized and proved that infections were caused by micro-organisms (and not by miasmic vapours in the air) and that a specific micro-organism was responsible for a specific disease. He pioneered as you well know the use of vaccines in the prevention of disease. There was also William Roentgen, a physicist who discovered X-rays, Marie Curie and her husband Pierre Curie, both physicists who discovered radium for the treatment of cancer, and Anton van Leeuwenhoek, who was not even a scientist, but a simple Dutch draper, whose curiosity and spirit of inquiry led to the discovery of the microscope.

Most universities in the West have a chair for the 'History of Medicine' and a curriculum on this subject for students entering medical school. I wish we could do likewise at least in some of our better known medical colleges and universities. I feel it is important for all medical students to know at least a little of the history of medicine, for it is only when you are aware of the past, that you will appreciate the present in its proper perspective.

Let me now briefly dwell on the present. Modern medicine to my mind starts with the discovery of penicillin by Alexander Fleming in 1928. For the first time in the history of medicine we had a drug which could effectively cure many potentially fatal infections. This discovery was the start of an antibiotic era which continues with the discovery of one antibiotic after another right up to the present day. Many other discoveries followed both in medicine and surgery—too numerous to detail; discoveries which would have been undreamt of just 50 years back. We live in the midst of these discoveries—a trifle aghast and staggered by their novelty and diversity encompassing not just medicine and surgery but all specialties. I will not even mention them because you are acquainted with them, you have learnt about them, and you are aware of their immense scope in the practice of medicine.

I will, however, briefly mention some features in relation to present-day medicine. We should to start with be humble enough to accept the fact that even today we have no absolute cure against some of the most common diseases afflicting mankind. We cannot cure hypertension, ischaemic heart disease, many forms of cancer, arthritis and mental diseases, to give just very few examples—we can alleviate these diseases, not cure them.

It is often forgotten when surrounded by a spate of dazzling modern discoveries, that nourishing food, hygiene, sanitation, clean drinking water and education, particularly of women, would go a long way to mitigate or even abolish a number of health problems faced by the poor developing countries of our world. Good medicine and the conquest of disease is thus inseparably linked with the socioeconomics of a country.

Please let not the science of medicine captivate you to the point where you forget its art. If you do so, you will imperil the doctor-patient relationship which is the very core of medicine. Compassion which breeds empathy towards your patient is the essence of medicine. If you lose this basic quality you may well become a cold calculating machine almost on par with the modern gadgetry that you will be using to investigate, monitor and treat your patient.

I would urge you to avoid expensive tests when simple tests suffice; weigh the cost-benefit ratio of whatever you do to your patient. Medical costs can impoverish both the patient and his or her family. Remember to communicate with your patients and with their relatives. Good communication is the secret of trust between the doctor and the patient. It is also one of the hallmarks of good patient care and reduces the risk of litigations that vitiate the path of modern medicine.

It is often forgotten that drugs and procedures can be hazardous—hazards that can be fatal. Risks and hazards are to an extent unavoidable in medicine and any drug or any procedure which is reasonably effective may have potential serious side-effects. It is important that you are always aware of this fact and that you are circumspect in their use.

I have always felt that as young doctors, you should know the basic important drugs in medicine very well, so that you become experienced and confident in their use. If in your practice you use a plethora of drugs, many of dubious value, you may do more harm than good. I am reminded of the famous saying of Oliver Wendell Holmes, 'I firmly believe that if the whole materia medica, as now used, were to be sunk to the bottom of the sea, it would be all the better for mankind—and all the worse for the fishes.'

This is of course an exaggeration, but is a reminder of the dangers that lurk behind the injudicious practice of medicine.

Finally, I need to remind you to be ethical in your practice. Contemporary medicine is both far-reaching and powerful, yet it harbours within itself, when incorrectly or inappropriately used, the potential to do harm. It is the cardinal principle of medical ethics that if you cannot do good, ensure that you do no harm. It is oft forgotten by the young, the inexperienced and the over-enthusiastic that in a number of medical and surgical problems, the need of the hour may warrant masterly inactivity rather than meddlesome interference. Also remember to respect your patient's right, the right to self-determination, the right after being properly informed, to refuse or accept medical investigations or treatment offered to him. In poor developing countries medicine cannot be divorced from socio-economic forces. When resources are limited as they inevitably are in most of our hospitals, justice demands that treatment is offered to patients who are most likely to benefit from them. This may often lead to an ethical quandary, impossibly difficult to solve.

Ours is a world of changing values where the finer qualities of life and living are increasingly being eroded by the lure of money and the acquisition of wealth. I would beseech you not to sacrifice your ethics, nor besmirch the virtue of your profession at the altar of greed or graft.

Let us now dream just a little of the future. The future really springs from the immediate past. It was the discovery of the structure of the DNA molecule by Watson and Crick in 1953 that has spawned the future. We will live in a century of rapidly advancing biotechnology, molecular biology and the science of genetics. They form the cutting edge of medicine today; they may well form the very core of medicine in the near future. Advances in reproductive physiology (sometimes of a frightening nature) will keep pace with advances in the science of genetics. We will live in a computer world with ever increasing strides made in information technology. These advances will knit the world closer and closer with time into one cohesive whole.

The human genome has already been deciphered. It is a matter of time before the precise biochemical code of each of the 100,000 genes is discovered. Genetic science should then determine how each gene functions and equally important, how a malfunctioning gene can influence or produce specific disease.

However, will all these advances make the world a happier place to live in? Will the burden of disease we carry with us today be significantly reduced? I do not expect the science of genetics to solve our major health problems. More than one gene may be responsible for the expression of common diseases like hypertension, diabetes, ischaemic heart disease and some forms of cancer. Again it is often the interaction between the gene and the environment which often determines the overt manifestations of a particular disease. The dangers of genetic engineering have been hotly debated. I dread the thought of genetic enhancement and genetic engineering changing Homo sapiens in the future to a species that would be unrecognizable to us today.

Advances in biotechnology, genetics and reproductive physiology will be chiefly the domain of the rich countries of the West. What of people in the continent of Africa and other poor countries, or for that matter even India? Will there be two classes of world citizens—those who enjoy the fruits of an increasingly powerful medicine of the future, and those who continue to struggle against disease with lesser means? The advances of genetic enhancement and genetic engineering if put to practical use may endow future citizens in developed countries with greater intelligence, powerful mental attributes, as also greater physical strength (perhaps the supermen and superwomen of the future!). Would not this dreadful class distinction lead to bitterness, strife, domination of one class over the other?

I look forward to the future with a mixture of hope and dread. Which path will medicine follow? What is its destination? Perhaps the future of medicine will be linked as in the past with philosophy, morals, ethics, economics and attitudes to life and living prevailing in centuries to come. I fear that if science captures medicine in its entirety, medicine will become increasingly cold, uncaring and even inhuman. In the not too distant past, all that the physician had to combat disease was courage, common sense, compassion and a few specific cures. Now that he has the awesome power of science and technology to back him, his human qualities will be increasingly on the wane. Is it not likely that the physician of the future will be embarrassed to hold the hand of a dying man, or tarry with him awhile to ease his passage into the unknown? The terrifying futuristic prospect of machines, computers and robots administering to the sick and suffering is matched by the even more terrifying concept of future man evolving as an appendage to a machine or evolving into half-machine, half-man. Hopefully this will not come to pass as mankind will reject such medicine as unworthy of its trust.

Will the concept of medicine change in the decades to come? Medicine from early centuries was built around changing models. Morgagni took the structure of an organ as the model of disease. Bichat took the tissue as his model. Virchow looked upon the cell as his model. Contemporary and future medicine have made the molecule as its model. This too will change in the near or distant future, for the history of science is the chronicle of change. Medicine in the future, will hopefully embrace the holistic model of the mind-body complex in which man is an integral part of nature. This will transpire when science proves that organs 'talk' to each other, communicate with and influence one another, to ensure that the human organism works as an integrated harmonious whole, vibrating in unison with nature. It will transpire when science proves that consciousness is a mysterious feature distinct from and unexplained by the anatomy and physiology of the billions of neurons that constitute the human brain. The control of the mind over the myriad functions of the body will then be elucidated as will the importance and use of bio-feedback mechanisms to influence the course of disease.

Finally, will science hand in hand with medicine solve the mystery of the nature of life and death? This is what Max Planck, one of the greatest physicists of the twentieth century has to say—'Science cannot solve the ultimate mystery of nature. And this is because in the final analysis we ourselves are part of nature and therefore part of the mystery we are trying to solve.'

Let me end by congratulating you on your academic achievements. Let me also thank you for your patient hearing. I wish you success in your profession and happiness in life. I must share with you some Oslerian advice. Concentrate on doing each day's work with all your might and forget the morrow, for the morrow will take care of itself. Be compassionate, caring and considerate to patients and colleagues. Cultivate a measure of equanimity. It will help you to bear the oft-felt agony of having to live among the sick, the dying and the dead; it will also enable you to withstand the vicissitudes of life with courage and fortitude.

When you set forth into the world, remember, 'The practice of medicine is an art, not a trade, a calling, not a business; a calling in which your heart will be exercised equally with your head'.

Euthanasia

It is not death I fear to face but dying.

—Robert Louis Stevenson

The word 'Euthanasia' is derived from the Greek word 'euthatos' (meaning 'good death'). A good death, a premeditated quick exit from the world has been a known practice from antiquity. The stoics took pleasure and pain, good fortune and misfortune with imperturbability, and chose death if they so wished, with the same calm and detachment they practised in life. The patrician Roman when the time came, was known to ask his slave, relative or friend to lay open his veins; he would then lie in a tub of warm water content to let his life slowly but surely ebb away. It was said to be a pleasant, dreamy exit from the world. Assisted suicide if one would like to call it, has often been practised as an act of compassionate duty on the field of battle. Tennyson embellished this concept when he wrote for Sir Richard Grenville aboard the battleship 'Revenge' at Flores in Azores.

Sink me the ship, Master Gunner–sink her, split her in twain!
Fall into the hands of God, not into the hands of Spain,
And the gunner said Ay Ay, but the seamen made reply,

We have childern, we have wives,
And the Lord has spared our lives.

'It was traditional, accepted because necessary, that some be set aside to die; by the surgeon in battle, the worst wounded; by the midwife at delivery, the unshapely born'. The field of battle is however not akin to the sick bed. In the modern context, euthanasia includes:

a) Voluntary euthanasia or intentional killing of patients who express a competent freely made wish to die because of the pain or suffering they experience;
b) Medically assisted suicide at the patient's insistence and wish;
c) Passive euthanasia in which doctors refrain from using devices to keep a terminally ill patient alive, or are even prepared to withdraw 'support' of various drugs or devices in those who are terminally ill;
d) Involuntary euthanasia where so-called mercy killing is perpetrated following a surrogate decision on a crippled or handicapped patient, or in a patient with a poor or even hopeless quality of life. In this case, the patient is not involved in the decision. Such an act truly amounts to homicide. To many, and in particular to theologists, this classification or differentiation is meaningless, for the forms described above are basically the same. It is the intention that defines the act and not the method used. Every 'method' stated above has the same intention—'to kill.'

The Question of Euthanasia

Euthanasia has been the subject of medical, political, ethical, religious and socioeconomic discussion in the West (particularly in the UK, Western Europe, North America) and in Australia for several decades. Voluntary euthanasia and physician-assisted suicide are now legal in the Netherlands, Belgium and in the American State of Oregon.

Euthanasia was legalized very briefly in the northern state of Australia. The debate on this subject is also slowly creeping into the developing countries such as India. However, the law as it stands in our country and in almost all countries is against all forms of euthanasia. The law is an ass, say the proponents and there are societies and groups in various countries determined to change the law. Why has there been such an increasing ferment, particularly in the West on euthanasia? The debate all over the world on this controversial issue was brought into increasingly sharp focus from the mid-seventies, ever since the tacit acceptance of euthanasia in the Netherlands and the toleration granted to it by the highest courts of this country. This ferment, this perturbation in Western society, particularly in the UK, US and Australia, continues undiminished to the present day. Remarkably enough, it is modern science and technology that have indirectly fuelled the debate. Fifty years ago, many seriously ill patients would have died within hours, days or at the most weeks. Today, medical skills, sophisticated gadgetry and ever increasing medical technology often prolong life even though death is inevitable, or support organ function even when personal identity is irrevocably and irretrievably lost. Again, patients not only in the West but also in India and other developing countries have developed an increasing independence of mind that counters the paternalistic dictates of doctors treating them. Many wish not to be 'kept alive' beyond a point, preferring to be allowed to die. In the West, some patients go even one step further and choose their time of dying requiring their doctors to bring about their death.

The attitude and approach of modern medicine towards not just the dying or the critically ill, but also to those unfortunate individuals who through illness, accident or defect have no sense of their personal identity, or are totally dependent, raise burning issues. The problem is not confined to medicine and to the doctor-patient relationship though this is indeed the focal point. There are ethical, religious, ideological, social and cultural overtones that strongly influence these burning issues. And of course there is the law—the law that considers the overall perspective and once laid down needs to be followed in the hope that a just, ordered society prevails.

I propose to briefly discuss these in relation to euthanasia. Obviously, my views are subjective, governed by my culture, personal beliefs, environment and upbringing—conditioned by my work as a physician over 50 years, many of which were spent in the care of the critically ill.

Ethical Principles in Medicine and their Relation to Euthanasia

The three ethical principles that govern a doctor-patient relationship are beneficence, autonomy and justice.

Beneficence directs the physician to do good by relieving suffering and restoring good health. Beneficence does not merely involve technical expertise and medical skill, it equally involves human qualities, particularly in the care of critically ill and terminally ill patients.

It is these human qualities which tend to be unfortunately forgotten or pushed into the background by the frontiers of advanced technology in medicine. The chief of these human qualities expressed as a single word is humanity. Humanity can be defined as the sensibility which enables a physician to feel for the distress and suffering of a patient, prompting him to relieve them. Knowledge and experience when linked to humanity make a great physician.

Non-maleficence is the companion-in-arms of beneficence. It reminds the physician that above all he should do no harm. 'Primum non nocere' (Above all do no harm). But those who clamour for euthanasia maintain that a doctor wilfully ending the life of a patient who expresses a competent wish to do so because of unbearable suffering or pain, is in fact practising an act of beneficence, of humanity and mercy.

I gather from discussions with my colleagues in the West, that a significant number of acutely ill patients who are about to die, as also patients with chronic but terminal disease express a desire to be killed or to be medically assisted in suicide. It is amazing that in my long association of close to 50 years, with so many critically ill patients in their terminal state, there has not been a single individual who has persistently wished for euthanasia. There have been a few who have expressed a fleeting wish, but talking to them and gently explaining measures to relieve their symptoms have led to a resigned and comparatively unanguished acceptance of their destiny. Why is there this difference between the East and the West? I think it is basically related to sociocultural and religious differences. A patient's and for that matter a physician's attitude to suffering, pain, impending death and death itself is conditioned by these sociocultural and religious factors. Most people in our part of the world and in the Far East tend to believe that life cannot be divorced from pain or suffering, that we live in the midst of pain and suffering, and that each one of us in this world is apportioned one's share of pain, and suffering. This is the law of 'karma'—a belief that one reaps in the present life what one has sown in previous lives, and that one will reap in future existences what one sows in the present.

The second basic ethical principle in medicine and in a doctor-patient relationship is patient autonomy. This is the patient's right to self-determination—the right after being properly informed to accept or refuse medical treatment offered to him including life-support measures like mechanical ventilation. It is indeed the proper interpretation of the balance between the principle of beneficence and the principle of patient autonomy that governs decision-making in medicine. The balance can be difficult and not easy to strike. This is because patients who are seriously ill may be unable to make proper decisions about their own care. In fact they may often make wrong or even absurdly perverse decisions under the physical and emotional stress of their illness. In these circumstances, particularly in acute problems and emergencies, when time is of essence, the physician in my opinion must lean towards the principle of beneficence and take management decisions which he genuinely believes are in the best interest of the patient.

The question therefore arises—should a doctor suppress his principle of beneficence at the altar of a patently perverse autonomous decision? Should he do so particularly in an acute situation when respecting this perverse autonomy would lead to certain death and countering it would almost certainly offer a restoration to a healthy life? My choice has been made clear; fear of the strict interpretation of the law might make colleagues in the West choose otherwise. Let me illustrate this dilemma with a few examples.

A woman of 26 years was brought to our critical care unit on the verge of death, with a note instructing that she was not to be resuscitated. The note was ignored (rightly or wrongly), resuscitation promptly started and after a difficult struggle the patient survived and was restored to perfect health. At discharge, she thanked and blessed the doctors for ignoring her note.

A married man of 30 years with two children and a caring wife was brought critically ill with a community-acquired pneumonia involving both lungs. He was in acute respiratory failure, cyanosed, very breathless, well nigh pulseless with a barely detectable blood pressure. He was on the verge of death and needed a ventilator to support his breathing and help oxygenate his blood. He refused the machine, in spite of my persuasion and also that of his family. We explained that his illness was reversible and that he had a good chance to return to perfect health. He held fast and persisted in his refusal. He was gasping and would have died within minutes if not promptly oxygenated. What was I to do? Was I not trained to heal, to help, to be beneficent? Again, rightly or wrongly (to my mind, quite rightly) we intubated him and kept him on ventilator support. He was too far gone at this point to resist. He was salvaged, recovered within a week, walked out of the unit with a smile, with profuse thanks and gifts for all the staff members!!

There are, however, times when patient autonomy conflicts with beneficence and is yet not necessarily patently perverse. It should be respected. For example, an elderly, seriously ill patient may make an informed well-considered directive that he would not submit to invasive procedures, or may refuse a biopsy or may refuse ventilator support or dialysis to support kidney function. Or he may refuse to be kept alive beyond a certain 'point'—again a legitimate autonomous decision. Patient autonomy is further strengthened in some countries of the West, as also in North America and Australia, by allowing a patient to give an advanced directive as to what he desires and what he does not desire in case of serious illness. This is acceptable to the Law and is commended to the medical profession in these countries. However, this advanced directive (also called The Living Will) can only forbid intervention or refuse consent to certain forms of treatment. It cannot issue a directive to any unlawful medical practice, so that direct killing or assisted suicide is untenable and against the law except in special circumstances, and that too only in those few countries where voluntary euthanasia and assisted suicide have been legalized.

The third and final ethical principle in medicine is justice—to distinguish the right from the wrong. If at times it is difficult or impossible to determine in absolute terms, one should determine what is more right or less wrong. Even in the West there is an ever increasing financial crunch for healthcare. Would it not be more just to expend resources on the ailing young who are useful to society and have a greater chance to survive than the very old who suffer dreadfully from chronic incurable illnesses or the terminally ill who clutter critical care units and hospital wards? Would not euthanasia in the terminally ill be beneficent and just? In developing countries where resources are even more limited, justice dictates that treatment is administered to patients who are most likely to benefit from it. This often produces an ethical quandary. Witness, for example, a situation where there are three ventilators in an eight-bedded tetanus ward, and all eight patients require mechanical ventilation. Physicians should unquestionably be involved in the ethics of resource distribution that provide equitable medical care to the society in which they live and work. Yet ethical arguments limiting care because of limited resources should not in my opinion be applicable to an individual patient already under care. Wisdom, however, dictates that in all situations requiring protracted care either in a critical illness or in a chronic incurable illness, the burden-benefit relationship should be carefully considered, and care be tempered with reason when judged to be an exercise in futility.

Euthanasia and the Intensive Care Unit

An intensive care unit (ICU) is a special unit that cares for critically ill patients who have potential for recovery. It also monitors patients whose symptoms and signs suggest that they may be on the verge of disaster. The unit is staffed by highly trained doctors, nurses and is supported by a network of trained technicians and health workers. The unit contains sophisticated gadgetry to closely monitor patients and to intervene often with invasive procedures or drugs in order to maintain and support deranged organ function. It is obvious that the unit has a high morbidity and mortality. There are no accurate figures in India, but in American and European studies mortality varied from 18-69 per cent, the variability being related to the case-mix in different units. In a UK study, of the patients who survived, only 58 per cent were alive two years after discharge from intensive care.

Is it possible to predict the outcome of critically ill patients in intensive care? Several studies have shown that the number of organs that fail to function adequately (organ dysfunction and failure) and the degree of organ failure determine mortality. The greater the number of organs that fail, the greater the mortality. Thus patients in whom more than three organs fail to function have a mortality of 85-100 per cent.

Many 'scoring systems' have been devised to predict the outcome and mortality in the ICU. Perhaps the most frequently used is the acute physiology and chronic health evaluation (APACHE) score. A score of 0-4 is assigned to each of the 11 measured physiological variables in a critically ill patient. It was shown that there is a predictable rise in mortality for each 5-point increase in this score. With a score of 5-9, the predicted mortality was 5-9 per cent. With a score greater than 35, the predicted mortality rose to 84 per cent. The APACHE score was developed by Knaus and colleagues at the George Washington University Center in a study of 5815 patients in 13 ICUs.

The question that arises is as follows—what should be the ethical approach to a patient who is dreadfully ill with an APACHE score suggesting an extremely high probability of death? A very high APACHE score (which is always associated with multiple organ dysfunction) merely predicts a very high risk of death for a large statistical group of patients. It does not predict the risk of death for individual patients. It is therefore patently wrong to 'abandon' such a patient or offer 'second-rate' treatment and care unless the patient has expressed a clear wish against certain procedures or certain modalities of treatment. Even then, as commented upon earlier, there may well be a clash between beneficence and patient autonomy which ethically is difficult to resolve. In our part of the world, multiple organ failure with high APACHE scores occurring in fulminant tropical infections do not carry the forbidding mortality reported in the ICUs in the West. This particularly applies to patients with fulminant plasmodium falciparum infection, a disease rampant in developing and tropical countries. It is a known fact that mortality in a critical illness is higher in the older age group (beyond 70 years). But the right to live is the first of all human rights and no other human right can exist without that human right. Also, the right to life exists irrespective of age, sex and race.

In my experience of over 40 years of work in a tertiary critical care unit, a number of patients who seemed on medical grounds very likely to die, ultimately survived, and were happy to be alive. It is true that many more equally ill patients failed to survive. But then does the doctor have the right to decide who should die and who should live?

There are a number of other ethical quandaries in the management of critically ill patients. I shall touch on a few of these by illustrative examples.

A 70-year-old patient with advanced cancer has at the most, three to six months to live. He is admitted to a critical care unit with an acute pneumonia. What is the ethical approach to the problem? One approach, often followed in the West is to leave him alone; let him have a quicker exit from this world because of the pneumonia. After all he has not long to live and even then what is the quality of his life? Often no question is asked of this patient as to what his views are to this approach.

The other view (and a view that I would follow) is to treat this patient for his pneumonia. An intensive care unit is meant to treat acute potentially reversible illness. If the patient survives, the patient himself and those close to him may value and even cherish the three to six months that he lives. And this indeed has often been so in my experience.

Let me give just one more example. An active, healthy man in his sixties was brought in comatose five years ago with a massive cerebral haemorrhage that had torn apart one cerebral hemisphere and ruptured into the ventricle and subarachnoid space. On admission and for some time after, even the basic brainstem reflexes were absent though an electroencephalogram (EEG) showed activity suggesting that he was not brain dead. It was explained to the relatives that the patient would almost certainly die, that recovery was well-nigh impossible, and even if by a miracle he recovered, he would be hopelessly crippled and handicapped. The relatives insisted that every effort should be made to treat him. All over the world, a patient such as this would have been allowed to die and our decision was likewise. But in India, though the patient comes first, the relatives for better or worse come a close second! It becomes very necessary to ascertain their views for social, cultural, and what is important for the treating doctor, for medicolegal reasons. When the relatives remained absolutely adamant and strongly antagonistic to our views, this patient was put on all medical support systems. After a long struggle, almost miraculously he survived. He was discharged in a conscious state, off all support systems after a month in the ICU and a month in the ward. His cognitive function improved further after another two months at home; his awareness of self returned as also his awareness of the environment and of those close to him. Today he moves about with support, communicates with relatives and friends, seems content, is glad to be alive in spite of his disability and is the joy of his wife, children and close friends.

A doctor can withhold treatment in an acute catastrophic illness if death seems certain. But it is often dangerous to withhold treatment based on the possible poor quality of life a patient is likely to experience with successful treatment. Who is to judge the quality of a patient's life? Again it is cultural and social differences between the East and the West that determine the attitude of doctors and patients to the deeper significance of life.

The Management of a Terminal Illness in the ICU

A terminal illness is one which is deemed incurable and in which death is inevitable. In the ICU, a terminal illness may last for a few hours to a few days. It is important in a given patient to review the word 'terminal' from hour to hour or day to day. Occasionally, what appears 'terminal' at one point offers hope after a lapse of time.

Patients judged 'terminal' by the treating doctor have been known to get well and go home! The responsibility of judging a patient as 'terminal' is therefore immense. At times the decision is easy and at times difficult. Clinical judgement, experience, wisdom are all involved in this decision. It may be impossibly difficult to decide when and where to draw the line. If there is even the slightest doubt it is better for all concerned to continue critical care and review events from time to time. Yet on a number of occasions the discerning physician can see the nearness and inevitability of death. The resource crunch in healthcare all over the world (particularly in our poor country) should prompt the physician in such a situation to refrain from using medical technology and skill that merely prolong death, or that makes death excessively lonely, gruesome, dehumanized, perhaps even obscene, and ruinous to the patient and family.

It is important in an acute illness which in spite of all efforts appears to progress to an inexorable fatal outcome to ascertain the wishes of the patient and his relatives. There is no document such as a Living Will in poor countries as there is in the West. Nevertheless there is still a very strong bond in our part of the world between the physician and the patient and the patient's relatives. The patient invariably follows the physician's advice and the relatives are similarly influenced. This is indeed an added and extremely heavy responsibility on the physician, because poor judgement can unnecessarily prolong the act of dying, and can also in the bargain financially cripple the patient's family. Better judgement could have prevented both these calamities. Judgement is terribly difficult in some young patients. Alas! It is not always that a Daniel comes to judgement.

A decision not to initiate invasive support, as for example the use of a ventilator or use of dialysis in a terminally ill patient is far more easy than the decision to withdraw support that has already been initiated at a point in time when the life-threatening acute illness seemed potentially reversible. A detailed discussion with relatives and close friends plays an important role in decision-making. Relatives need to accept when intensive care is futile and when support in all forms is either not initiated or withdrawn. Withdrawing support in all forms when death is close and inevitable is increasingly practised not only in the Western world but also in India, not withstanding the legal issues raised in our country.

Management of a terminal illness in the ICU is further helped by the following principles:

1) The proper training of doctors, nurses and students in the management of terminal illness, with special reference to palliative care briefly discussed later.
2) The offering of true compassion to the patient—a quality which can neither be bought or taught, but which should come naturally to all well-trained staff in good centres.

Palliative Care

The answer to the management of terminal illness in the ICU or of terminally ill patients (at home, in hospital or in a hospice) due to a chronic incurable illness does not lie in voluntary euthanasia or patient-assisted suicide, but the practice of palliative care, which includes the practice of palliative medicine. The latter has now become a speciality with protocols to deal with various physical and emotional vicissitudes encountered in the terminally ill. Pain control has evolved far beyond the mere administration of opiates, opiate derivatives and sedatives. Yet in poor countries these drugs still remain the sheet anchor of pain control. Many doctors, nurses and health workers fail to use an appropriate dose of opiates or their derivatives for fear of depressing respiration and circulation, thereby endangering life or hastening death. In this connection, a quote from a judgment delivered in the UK by Judge Delvin is indeed of unsurpassed guidance and relevance—'The proper medical treatment that is administered and that has an incidental effect in determining the exact moment of death, is not the cause of death in any sensible use of the term.'

The World Health Organization (WHO) defines palliative care as follows—The active total care of patients whose disease is not responsive to curative treatment. Control of pain or other symptoms and of psychological, social and spiritual problems is paramount. The goal of palliative care is the achievement of the best possible quality of life for the patient and the family.

Palliative medicine is comparatively cheap and can be offered at home, in hospital or in the hospice. It respects life and considers death as a natural inevitable sequel. When correctly practised it does not protract the act of dying nor generally hasten it. It helps support the patient in the transition from life to death and lends support and comfort to those close to the patient during this period of treatment. Palliative medicine when practised with an equal measure of skill and compassion should hopefully render the current commotion and debate on euthanasia in the West both obsolete and redundant.

Euthanasia in relation to the Persistent Vegetative State, Alzheimer's Disease and related Dementias

A persistent vegetative state (PVS) is a rare entity characterized by the preservation of brainstem reflexes but with total loss of cortical function due to damage to the neocortex. It is generally caused by prolonged deprivation of oxygen to the brain (hypoxia). There is a total loss of conscious awareness, a total loss of cognition, loss of all emotional response, loss of all movements and a total obliteration of every feature of personality. Patients in a persistent vegetative state appear to be awake with their eyes open, but do not respond to visual, tactile or auditory stimuli. They generally breathe normally, have a normal circulatory system but are hopelessly dependent. They need to be fed through a nasogastric tube and they have no control over the bladder or the bowels. When cared for, these patients can continue in this vegetative state for years.

What is the ethical approach to this rare medical problem? It may
be impossible for several reasons for such a patient to be cared for
at home by family members. If so, is a state-funded hospital obliged
to care for this patient indefinitely? To what extent should this care
be offered? The medical moral, ethical, legal issues involved and the
solutions offered are perhaps and only perhaps illustrated by a rather
unique case of PVS which was deliberated upon by the highest court
in the United Kingdom.

Anthony Bland in 1989 suffered a crush-injury to his chest and lung
in the Hillsborough Stadium disaster. In spite of all medical efforts
he evolved over months into a PVS due to irreversible damage to his
cerebral cortex caused by cerebral hypoxia. He showed no signs of
improvement or arousal over the next three and a half years. The
health authority responsible for the hospital caring for him appealed
to the court for permission to discontinue procedures (including the
use of nasogastric feeds to maintain nutrition) that had been required
to preserve his life. The High Court in a judgment stated that it was
indeed permissible to do so. In December 1992 the Court of Appeal
in England considered an appeal against this judgment and ruled that
the medical staff caring for the patient should be judged as acting
within the law if they discontinued life-sustaining measures (also
discontinuing nasogastric feeds) for Anthony Bland. This decision of
the Court of Appeal was upheld by the House of Lords in what is
considered a landmark judgment. The judgment of Lord Hoffman
carries great legal, ethical, and intellectual authority. I prefer, however,
to quote the relevant part of this judgment because of the clarity with
which his Lordship discriminated ethically and legally, valid forms of
management from the forms of management which were invalid, in
relation to those unfortunate patients imprisoned permanently into a
state of mental and emotional, non-being or nothingness. I quote,

'In my view, the choice which the law makes must reassure people
that the courts do have full respect for life, but that they do not
pursue the principle to the point at which it has become almost

empty of any real content and when it involves the sacrifice of other important values such as human dignity and freedom of choice. I think that such reassurance can be provided by a decision, properly explained to allow Anthony Bland to die. It does not involve, as the counsel for the Official Solicitor suggested a decision that he may die because the court thinks that his life is not worth living. There is no question of his life being worth living or not worth living because the stark reality is that Anthony Bland is not living a life at all. None of the things that one says about the way people live their lives well or ill, with courage or fortitude, happily or sadly—have any meaning in relation to him. This in my view represents a difference in kind from the case of the conscious but severely handicapped person. It is absurd to conjure up the spectre of eugenics as a reason against the decision in this case.

Thus, in principle I think it would be right to allow Anthony Bland to die. Is this answer affected by the proposed manner of his death? Some might say that as he is going to die, it does not matter how. Why wait for him to expire for lack of food or be carried off by an untreated infection? Would it not be more human to give him a lethal injection? No one in this case is suggesting that Anthony Bland should be given a lethal injection. But there is concern about ceasing to supply food as against, for example, ceasing to treat an infection with antibiotics. Is there any real distinction? In order to come to terms with our infinitive feelings about whether there is a distinction, I must start by considering why most of us would be appalled if he was given a lethal injection. It is, I think, connected with our view that the sanctity of life entails its inviolability by an outsider. Subject to exceptions like self-defence, human life is inviolate even if the person in question has consented to its violation. That is why although suicide is not a crime, assisting someone to commit suicide is. It follows that, even if we think Anthony Bland would have consented we would not be entitled to end his life with a lethal injection.

On the other hand, we recognize that one way or another, life must come to an end. We do not impose on outsiders an unqualified duty to do everything possible to prolong life as long as possible. I think that the principle of inviolability explains why, although we accept that in certain cases it is right to allow a person to die (and the debate so far has been over whether this is such a case) we hold without qualification that no one may introduce an external agency with the intention of causing death. I do not think that the distinction turns upon whether what is done is an act or omission. The distinction is between an act of omission which allows an existing cause to operate and the introduction of an external agency of death.'

The following four points in this judgment stand out in sharp focus. First, it is absolutely not permissible on ethical and legal grounds to take life in the terminal stage, or any stage of any patient's illness, whatever the physical or mental state. We need to uphold and practise not just respect but show reverence for life. Dr Albert Schweitzer expresses this beautifully in his autobiography. 'The ethics of reverence for life therefore comprehends within itself everything that can be described as love, devotion and sympathy. It is in fact the essence of all Christianity and the essence of all religions. In fact it is a religion in itself.'

Second, there is a qualitative difference between killing on intent and allowing the process of dying to take its natural course. Those who disregard the above two principles could only serve to shatter the doctor-patient relationship and the trust patients repose in the medical profession. They would perhaps best be termed executioners rather than healers. One needs only to remember the Nazi era of the previous century when even doctors among so many others stifled their conscience into non-existence so that habitual killing progressed to mass murder of the innocents. One needs also only remember the dreadful exploits of Dr Kevorkian who perhaps thought that he was the pioneer of a brave, new, benign medical world that needed to kill the aged, the infirm, handicapped and dependent, because they were presumably (so he thought) miserable in the quality of their lives, burdensome, expensive to maintain, eating into a large chunk of an ever increasing healthcare budget. If the first two points deduced from Lord Hoffman's judgment were to be flouted or in years to come overturned, it would not be too far-fetched to envision a society that practised Kevorkianism in the name of charity, humanity and convenience!

The third point that comes into focus is that patients who are unconscious, oblivious of their own self, to persons and the world around them, and insensate to either pain or pleasure, have no life to live. They therefore need to be protected from further erosion of their integrity by being allowed to die.

The fourth and last point is that in such a situation cessation of medical treatment and artificial feeding should be considered as neither illegal or unethical.

I am in no position to dispute this judgment. I shall, however, illustrate my ethical quandary with regard to the third and fourth points of Lord Hoffman's judgment by briefly describing a patient presently under my care.

A lady of 65 years suffered hypoxic brain damage and in spite of all attempts progressed to a PVS. She has been in this state for over two years and there is absolutely no hope for improvement. She has an only daughter who even in her mother's present state, loves her to distraction. The daughter works the whole day with an advertising firm and comes every night to the hospital to visit her. She speaks into her ear and often sings to her. When repeatedly explained that her mother is oblivious to her own self, to her and all that she says, she just replies with an enigmatic smile on her caring face. She keeps a day and night nurse to look after the mother and would be devastated even if a suggestion is made that we should now let her be. We all look after the mother as well as we look after our other patients. She is fed by a nasogastric tube, has a tracheostomy tube (an artificial airway) to keep her airways open, and a urinary catheter to drain her bladder. She has occasional infections, some of which we ignore and some we treat, particularly if she runs high fever. We have refrained from invasive monitoring or any form of invasive support. How can we ever convince the daughter that the correct approach is to let her mother go? How could we even suggest that we stop feeding her? It would shatter the daughter if we did not look after her mother. A doctor's duty (medical and ethical) is to the patient, but must he not take the wishes of someone as close to the patient as this daughter?

The third and fourth points of Lord Hoffman's judgment in my opinion do not apply to other dementias and to Alzheimer's disease. It is only in the very last stages of Alzheimer's disease that patients have no cognition and even then the physical and mental state differ subtly from those seen in patients suffering from a PVS. It would be prudent not to use invasive procedures as far as possible in these conditions, but it would be ethically justifiable and correct to treat infections which are reversible and to continue to feed them.

It is also extremely important for care givers—doctors, nurses and other health professionals to give the same medical attention and treatment to the medically handicapped as to those who are mentally competent. The medically handicapped have the same right to live as anyone else in the world.

Not uncommonly, medical decisions on the demented or in those physically and mentally disabled are made with reference to their presumed quality of life. This has already been alluded to earlier, but a few further comments are necessary. It is not fair for a doctor or for any other person to pass judgement on the quality of life of a patient. The acid test is how the patient feels and reacts to what he feels. It is amazing to see patients who to us seem to have intolerable defects, cope with them with aplomb and good cheer. It is also amazing how people in good health who pity and deprecate the poor quality of life in a disabled friend or relative exhibit the same good cheer and aplomb when struck by a disease that results in an even worse disability.

Management decisions in patient care are also at times based on the 'patient's best interest'. One often hears a statement to this effect—it is in the best interests (of a mentally or physically handicapped patient) that infection remains untreated or that nasogastric feeds be stopped. Even if these decisions are valid under certain circumstances, a patient oblivious to his surroundings, or severely handicapped, is either not aware of his interest or perhaps unable to express his interest. Therefore, not uncommonly, decisions such as these are being made to please others and not made in the best interests of the patient.

Euthanasia and the Law

Besides the countries mentioned earlier, Germany and Switzerland have also legalized physician-assisted suicide but not voluntary euthanasia. It was the Netherlands that in a way set the ball rolling. I shall briefly describe how euthanasia came about in this country. It all started with a landmark decision of the Netherlands Supreme Court in 1984 on the Alkmaar case. This case concerned a 95-year-old lady who was incurably ill and who made repeated requests to her doctor to put an end to her unbearable suffering. The doctor acceded to the request. The doctor was convicted by the Court of Appeals at Amsterdam but the conviction was set aside and the doctor was acquitted by the Supreme Court and the Court of the Hague. The only reason for acquittal accepted by the Supreme Court was the invocation of a situation of force majeure (or necessity) arising from a conflict of duties—the duty to preserve a patient's life and the duty to alleviate unbearable suffering. If taking into consideration the special circumstances of the case, a doctor has balanced these conflicting duties before making a decision that can be objectively justified, he stands acquitted.

In the same year the Royal Dutch Medical Association issued a statement on euthanasia stating that voluntary euthanasia was acceptable under certain circumstances. They formulated a set of criteria with safeguards in its practice. These criteria mirror the criteria developed by the courts—

- The request for euthanasia must come from the patient; it should be entirely voluntary, persistent, well-considered.
- The patient must experience intolerable pain or suffering (physical or mental) with no acceptable solutions to alleviate the situation.
- Euthanasia must be performed after consultation with a colleague experienced in the field.

Other questions addressed by the courts in subsequent decisions were as follows:

A patient's request in the form of an advanced directive drawn up by the patient when still competent was valid and to be respected.

The courts did not require that a patient is terminally ill nor does it require that death is imminent. They also ruled that unbearable suffering need not only be physical; it could also be psychological. Euthanasia was tolerated and granted protection in all these events, if the patient was in an untenable situation and no alternatives were available.

In 1985, the State Commission on Euthanasia appointed to advise the Netherlands government on future legislation, proposed that voluntary euthanasia should not be considered an offence if carried out by a doctor on a patient who makes a specific request for it, provided the patient was in an untenable situation with no prospect of improvement. The proposal to amend the Dutch Penal Code to this effect did not however succeed.

It was an accepted fact that unregulated covert euthanasia was practised by doctors and nurses not only in the Netherlands but in several countries of the world. The deliberations of the Royal Dutch Medical Association, the recommendations of the State Commission and above all the pattern of court rulings that offered protection to the practice of euthanasia under very special circumstances served to bring this covert practice out into the open for discussion and debate. How frequent was this covert practice? The Remmelink Commission was set up by the State government to determine data not only on the practice of euthanasia in the Netherlands, but also on other medical decisions concerning the end of life, such as withdrawing or withholding treatment. The results of this survey have been discussed later.

All through the nineties of the last century, euthanasia was not legalized in the Netherlands, despite the recommendations and the court rulings. Yet a balance was struck between statutory law that prohibited euthanasia and case laws which laid down specific circumstances and conditions for non-prosecution and permitted its controlled acceptance in practice. Ultimately the pressure to change the law became irresistible; and in April 2002 both voluntary euthanasia and physician-assisted suicide finally became legal in the Netherlands — the first country to allow doctors to put an end to the life of patients who had 'unbearable suffering'. The new law insists that the patients must be above 12 years (patients between 12 and 16 years of age required the consent of the parents).

Doctors involved in voluntary euthanasia or suicide must:

a) be convinced that the patient's request was voluntary, well-considered and lasting;
b) be convinced that the patient's suffering was unremitting and unbearable;
c) have informed the patient of the situation and prospects;
d) have reached the conclusion with the patient that there was no reasonable alternative;
e) have consulted at least one other physician;
f) have carried out the procedure in a medically appropriate fashion.

(Section 293 (2) Of the Dutch Criminal Code)

Belgium and the State of Oregon in the US followed suit with similar legislation. Many other countries have been the target of significant reformist pressure but the courts and legislators have so far been firm and have refused to remove the fundamental criminal law objection to euthanasia and to assisted suicide. In the West, the North American continent, Australia and New Zealand, legal sanction has been granted to withhold or withdraw treatment under special circumstances. A similar practice quietly prevails in many other tertiary units all over the world not withstanding the lack of legal sanction. Problems will arise when this right has to be exercised on behalf of incompetent patients. Constitutional liberty and equality rights have been involved in both the US and Canada to challenge criminal law proceedings on assisted suicide. The courts so far have rejected these arguments.

The concept and the use of advanced directives (living will) is increasingly accepted in many counties in the West. Judicial comments point to a sympathetic attitude towards such statements of preference. Yet living wills can often be ambiguous and the question often arises whether an earlier statement necessarily reflects the current view of a patient.

In India, euthanasia in any form is illegal. Brain death is recognized but support systems can only be taken off and the patient declared dead, if the patient concerned has consented to be a donor for any organ transplant. If not, death occurs legally only when the heart, circulation and respiration cease.

Though in many ICUs, under special circumstances, treatment may be withheld or withdrawn, (and this holds true in many tertiary centres in many countries of the world), to the best of my knowledge there is no legal sanction for this in India. For example, if a patient is on mechanical ventilator support, there is no legal sanction to withdraw this support till death occurs even if a competent doctor feels that such support in a given circumstance merely protracts the act of dying. Finally, though a right to patient autonomy is recognized there is no legal validity or legal weightage (as far as I know) to advanced directives or a living will in India.

The Debate—The Heart of the Matter

The law in almost all countries of the world has so far stood steadfastly against euthanasia. Undoubtedly, belief in the sanctity of life enshrined in the teachings of all great religions of the world is central to this decision. In India and many poor developing countries, religion, philosophy and culture lend even greater strength to the law on this subject. But will the belief in the sanctity of life always hold? We live in a world of changing values, where consumerism, market forces and self-gratification play overriding roles. We live in an evidence-based world of science so that faiths and beliefs even when encrusted by age and tradition are no longer accepted and come into question. The emphasis is a demand for 'rights', not the acceptance of duties. The 'right to die with dignity' and to legalize euthanasia are slogans often linked together as if one needs the latter to achieve the former. Amazingly, in my long experience, those (at least in India) who championed most vociferously the 'right to die with dignity' suffered protracted, incurable illnesses without a whisper or a whimper!

The Right to Die

The right to life is protected by the law. Even if the belief in the sanctity of life is forgotten, the belief in the respect for life remains universal in all civilized societies. The right to life is basic, inalienable, unqualified. An imbecile has the same right as a genius, a newborn the same as a centenarian, one suffering from a terminal illness or one hideously malformed has the same right as one in his prime. But is there a right to die? And even if this be so, can one extend that right to allow another individual to execute that right or at least aid and abet in its fruition? No such right is articulated (to the best of my knowledge) in the constitution of any country or in the Declaration of Human Rights, or the European Convention on Human Rights yet it is this claim to the 'right to die' that fuels the argument for the change in law on euthanasia.

Medical practice bristles with difficulties when patients (not terminally ill) either refuse treatment or insist on withdrawal of treatment that is life-giving or life-sustaining. Not only is there a conflict between patient autonomy and beneficence—the two basic principles that govern the doctor-patient relationship, but there is also the ethical and legal difficulty in interpreting such refusals. I shall give a few illustrative examples. A patient with cancer may refuse surgery which could cure him knowing full well the consequences of his choice. His refusal is respected by the law. In law, an imposition of unwanted therapy constitutes assault, even if the doctors genuinely believe that the patient will benefit from it. Under these circumstances, would the patient's refusal be considered an expression of his right to die? Or is it merely a 'choice' which does not necessarily amount to a 'right'? This is a subtle question for the legal profession.

There have been an increasing number of judgments in the West over the last 15 years when the court has granted permission for the removal of a ventilator essential to support life in a totally paralyzed patient who is *not* terminally ill, but in whom recovery is judged to be impossible. Even if this is done at the patient's specific, persistent request and consent, does such a judgment indirectly construe that the patient has a right to die? Or could one say that the judgment was tantamount to an 'aid' to suicide? Judgments in similar circumstances have not been uniform, illustrating the unresolved moral and legal complexities of this problem.

The practice of euthanasia in the Netherlands is being keenly followed by the world at large. How does it fare? What does it reveal? The results of a survey of this practice undertaken by the Remmelink Commission during 1990-91 are pertinent. There were 2300 cases of voluntary euthanasia in 1990 with a further 400 cases of physician-aided suicide. Amazingly, the maximum requests for euthanasia in this survey were related to either a 'loss of dignity' or 'being dependent on others' or being 'tired of life' rather than to just physical suffering and pain. These requests were acceded to by doctors under protection of the law. Many would find this shocking. It is the old, lonely, dependent and poor who have little or no access to curative or palliative care. It is this vulnerable section of society that needs to be protected. Not to do so is not to value life, to negate the first and most basic of all human rights—the right to life. I firmly believe that 'respect for human life, even if it allows an individual to choose to end that life demands that no third party should usurp that choice'.

It was also noted by the Remmelink Commission that doctors terminated the life of an additional 1000 patients by the administration of drugs without the patient's explicit consent or request. Could not the practice of covert involuntary euthanasia (which is homicide or manslaughter, according to the law) multiply a thousandfold or even a millionfold if the law was not doubly vigilant? Though the patients were reported to be terminally ill, this practice could surreptitiously be extended to the most dependent and vulnerable in society. We again need to remember the Nazi regime in the last century to realize that this is not an impossible exaggeration.

In the East the law against euthanasia is almost certain to remain sacrosanct in the foreseeable future. I cannot offer an expert comment on what the future holds for the West. Changing values, social pressures, soaring, impossible-to-meet costs of healthcare, difficulties in offering palliative care to an ever increasing ageing population, may all shape the law differently. However, to the fore, will always remain the increasingly strident plea that the relief of unbearable unmitigated suffering through euthanasia is an act of beneficence and an act of humanity. Such a plea strikes a sympathetic emotional chord in an increasing number of decent well-meaning people in the world. If the law does change it will undoubtedly do so under strict clauses and safeguards. But can the law effectively police the boundary between an act of beneficence which humanely ends suffering from an act manifesting a total disregard for life? Would not the fear of covert compulsion instead of explicit wish and consent, haunt the practice of euthanasia? In spite of all safeguards and guarantees, is it not possible that a patient may want to end his suffering as a matter of a cult, or even as a matter of duty to relatives and friends? Will it ever be possible to quantify suffering? Can most doctors claim to have the knowledge, the experience, the Oslerian wisdom and perspective to be truly able to enlist themselves in the cause of euthanasia in a patient who states ' I cannot bear the suffering I am going through'? These are pertinent questions difficult to answer. Finally, when one legalizes a solution to a problem like euthanasia, would the good that accrues clearly outbalance the evil or harm that could conceivably result from this legal sanction? This indeed is the heart of the matter.

Landmarks in Modern Medicine

A great discovery is a fort whose appearance in science gives rise to shining ideas, whose light dispels many obscurities and shows us new paths.

—CLAUDE BERNARD

The history of medicine is an epic of splendid human endeavour and achievement. The advances and discoveries of modern medicine in particular, are truly epochal and will remain as indelible landmarks in the history of man. A citizen in any part of the world living in the early twentieth century would have considered the present medical scene and achievements unthinkable—medical fiction, a figment of a fervid imagination. This is because modern medicine has made a dramatically successful assault on many previously untreatable diseases and has come up with a spate of discoveries producing a tremendous impact on man.

Let me list some of the landmark discoveries of modern medicine that have brought benefit to mankind. Antibiotics are capable of curing many previously untreatable diseases; the scourge of smallpox has been wiped off the surface of the earth; poliomyelitis has been conquered except in a few poor countries. Therapeutic advances can control hypertension, diabetes, heart diseases, asthma, inflammatory and degenerative diseases of the joints, many forms of cancer and several other problems that afflict the mind and body. The discovery of cortisone for the treatment of rheumatoid arthritis unwittingly heralded the control of several other unrelated diseases, cutting across a gamut of different specialities. Open heart surgery, organ transplants, joint replacements, laparoscopic diagnosis and laparoscopic surgery are other major advances that have helped a vast number of people. Advances in reproductive physiology led to the discovery of the contraceptive pill, which in a way liberated women, and then to the realization of *in vitro* fertilization and test-tube babies. Landmarks in diagnostics include advances in imaging techniques—ultrasound, high-resolution computerized tomography, magnetic resonance imaging and positron emission tomography (PET) scanning. The structure of deoxyribonucleic acid (DNA) which in fact is the biochemistry of life and existence, was unravelled around the middle of the twentieth century laying open the hitherto unexplored vista of genetic medicine. The human genome was deciphered to its minutest details in 2000. The impact of the last two discoveries not just on medicine, but on life, living and perhaps even on the evolution of the human race is yet to be felt. There is no field of medicine which has escaped the strong impact of modern medicine.

To detail all these and many other advances would require volumes. I have chosen to write briefly on just three of these landmark discoveries in modern medicine. My choice is arbitrary, influenced perhaps by the need to bring to the reader the fortuitousness of some great discoveries, the role played by circumstances and good fortune, together with the importance of astute observation, single-minded determination and devotion in pursuing an objective to a successful end.

Before I do so, when does modern medicine actually start? To review the landmarks of modern medicine we must gaze not just at the immediate present but necessarily look at the recent past. Is there a dividing line, a watershed in medicine between the 'old' and what is modern or 'new'? There probably is, but the 'new' is built upon the 'old'; the wonders of modern medicine would have never been realized had they not been preceded by even earlier discoveries. Unfortunately, we live in an era which has its focus on 'what is', the immediate present, as also on 'what is to be'—the future. Is it therefore worthwhile to give the reader a glimpse of the recent past? I do believe so, for the past in any field of endeavour permeates the present and lies buried within the future. 'The historical sense involves the perception not only of the pastness of the past but of its presence'(T.S. Eliot). To gain a proper perspective, the never-ending canvas of medicine is best viewed in its entirety—the past, the present, the changing unfinished future.

I would date modern medicine 25 to 30 years after the start of the twentieth century. The therapeutic advances and discoveries that have conferred the greatest benefit to mankind originate and follow from that period of time. It is of interest to know what medicine was before this date. Well past the middle of the nineteenth century, medical therapy for diseases was to either purge, starve or bleed the patient no matter what he suffered from. More deaths perhaps occurred from the ministrations of the physician than from the disease itself. There were just a few drugs of proven efficacy. There was digitalis derived from the foxglove plant discovered by William Withering for heart disease, quinine derived from the cinchona bark brought back to Europe by Jesuits from South America for the treatment of malaria, salicylates obtained from the bark of the willow tree, used for rheumatic fever, colchicine useful for gout, and opium, the most widely used drug for relief of pain or of suffering in any form. Jenner had discovered vaccination against smallpox; this was followed by immunization of varying effectiveness against other infectious diseases. The early 1900s saw the discovery of vitamins for treatment of vitamin deficiency diseases, the discovery of thyroxine for hypothyroidism, the discovery of insulin for the treatment of diabetes, the use of salversan (an arsenical compound) for the specific treatment of syphilis and the introduction of sulphonamides to treat infections.

It was, however, the discovery of penicillin by Alexander Fleming in 1929 that heralded the avalanche of therapeutic discoveries that followed. Arbitrary as it unquestionably is, I would consider this the first landmark discovery in modern medicine. Why should I consider it so? For the first time in the history of man and medicine we had a drug which could treat and cure many acute often fatal infections—pneumonia, meningitis, bacterial sepsis, just to name a few. It also helped to treat and cure chronic infections affecting the sinuses, joints, skin and to successfully fight venereal disease such as syphilis and gonorrhea.

Penicillin (termed an antibiotic) was the by-product of a fungus penicillium occurring in nature. Its discovery stimulated a search for similar substances to fight infections; it opened up an era of antibiotic discovery which continues to the present day. It raised the hopes and aspirations of both man and medicine. Could there not in the near future be similar discoveries for the treatment of other dreaded diseases, such as heart ailments, hypertension, cancer or of mental illnesses such as schizophrenia? The discovery of penicillin was therefore indeed a magical moment in the history of modern medicine. Let us relive this magical moment.

Alexander Fleming was a brilliant student who wished to become a surgeon. However, in 1906, with the intention of staying in the hospital rifle-shooting squad, he took a temporary job in the Innoculation Department headed by the famous scientist Sir Almroth Wright, at St. Mary's Hospital, London. This was a quirk of destiny for Fleming and for the world. He took up bacteriology, discovered penicillin in 1928 and stayed on at St. Mary's for 49 years.

During the First World War, Fleming worked on wounds, infection in wounds and resistance to infection. He noted that chemical agents used to clean wounds damaged the natural defences, failing to kill the bacteria responsible for infection. His first important discovery was the discovery of an enzyme present in tears and mucous fluids. He called this enzyme lysozyme because of its ability to lyse organisms contaminating a culture of nasal mucus. He regarded lysozyme as part of the natural defences of the body against infection.

In 1928, Fleming started his work on the bacteriology of staphylococci, dangerous pus-forming organisms, often contaminating wounds and frequently responsible for abscesses, fatal sepsis and septicaemia. Returning from a three-week holiday, he noted that one of the Petri dishes growing staphylococci had been contaminated by mould spores and that the bacteria near that mould had been destroyed. The mould spores could have come in through an open window, though it is more probable that they floated up the stairs from a laboratory below, where a researcher was investigating fungi. Fleming could have just thrown the Petri-dish away as 'contaminated'! He did not; he was intrigued, he researched further, identifying the mould as Penicillium. He made the discovery that a powerful antibiotic substance had seeped out of the Penicillium and killed the staphylococci. He called this antibiotic penicillin. He believed that the mould responsible for secreting penicillin was *Penicillium rubrum*. In fact it was later shown to be *Penicillium notatum*. His further work proved that penicillin was effective against gram-positive cocci like streptococci, pneumococci, meningococci, gonococci, staphylococci but not against gram-negative organisms. He also noted that the antibiotic did not adversely affect healthy tissues or leucocyte function. Fleming and the scientific world now forgot about this discovery. He failed to take the next obvious step of using penicillin in animals deliberately innoculated with gram-positive pathogenic bacteria. This lapse is amazing and was probably due to his observation that when penicillin was mixed with blood in a laboratory, it lost its efficacy. He failed to realize that what happens in a test-tube in a laboratory could not necessarily be equated with what happens in a human body. In 1929, Fleming published his work on the discovery of penicillin and turned his attention to other research.

Remarkably enough other scientists could not replicate Fleming's findings when they experimented by dropping penicillium mould onto an agar plate studded with colonies of staphylococci. It was not until 1964 that the reason for this became obvious. Robert Hare, Fleming's former assistant who investigated the matter in depth, explained that the failure to replicate Fleming's original observation was because the penicillium mould grew best at a temperature of 20° C and the staphylococcus grew best at a temperature of 35° C. To start with the penicillium mould (*Penicillium notatum*) that probably floated upward through the window from the laboratory of a fellow scientist studying fungi, was a rare strain that produced large amounts of penicillin. Some spores of this fungus presumably contaminated the Petri dish on which Fleming had grown colonies of staphylococci. For some inexplicable reason, Fleming before proceeding for his holiday had left the Petri dish on the bench rather than in the incubator. Robert Hare, consulting meteorological records for London at the end of July 1929, observed that when Fleming was away, London went through an exceptionally cool nine-day period that could have favoured a vigorous growth of the penicillium mould. This was followed by a rise in temperature which could have favoured the growth of staphylococci. The penicillium mould in the cold nine-day period could have produced sufficiently large quantities of penicillin. On his return Fleming noted that for a considerable distance surrounding the mould, colonies of staphylococci had undergone lysis—that is they had been destroyed. Thus without the nine-day cool period towards the end of July 1929, which stimulated a vigorous growth of the penicillium mould (which secreted larger quantities of penicillin), Fleming would not have discovered penicillin!

The discovery of penicillin would have remained buried in the archives of medical journals had it not been for a brilliant Australian pathologist, Howard Florey. Howard Florey headed the Dunn School of Pathology at Oxford, at the young age of 37. In 1935 he hired biochemist Ernst Chain, a German Jew who had just escaped from the Nazis. The two teamed up and began a search for a powerful antibacterial substance. After going through over 200 papers they came across the work of Fleming. Florey and Chain grew *Penicillium notatum*, but encountered great difficulties in isolating the active ingredient from the liquid produced by the mould. Only one part in two million was pure penicillin. Perhaps they might have given up, had it not been for Norman Heatley, another biochemist in the team. Heatley devised techniques to improve the yield of penicillin and of purifying it.

The Second World War had commenced, but this work went on despite lack of funds and equipment and the risk of German air raids. On Saturday, 25 May 1940, Florey and his colleagues innoculated eight mice with lethal doses of streptococci; four were then given penicillin. By 1.45 am the next morning, the mice that had not received the drug had died, but the four who had received the penicillin were alive and well. Florey exulted, 'It looks like a miracle'.

The mice experiments had been done at a critical phase of the Second World War. France was on the verge of defeat and the British expeditionary force driven to the beaches of Dunkirk were being evacuated by an armada of ships that survived the onslaught of the Luftwaffe. Florey, Chain and Heatley, however, realized the great potential of penicillin to treat infections and in particular war wounds. Florey decided to convert his department into a manufacturing plant to make penicillin. This decision was a courageous one; had it failed it could have invited strong censure. It involved committing all funds and resources of his department to this project; it necessitated continuous hard work from not only the scientists but from other colleagues in his department. Shortage of funds and the weight of urgent necessity led to remarkable improvization. Heatley found that the best receptacles for growing penicillium mould were sterilized bed-pans. These sterilized bed-pans were coated with culture medium, sprayed with penicillium spores through spray guns, then wheeled into a students' preparation room converted into a huge incubator at 24° C. The fluid from these moulds was then extracted and stored in milk jugs!

At last Florey thought that there was enough penicillin to try on a human patient. Albert Alexander was a policeman who developed staphylococcal sepsis and multiple abscesses all over his body following a scratch on his face sustained while pruning roses. Charles Fletcher was the doctor who on 12 February 1941 administered penicillin intravenously every three hours to this patient. The patient's urine was collected over 24 hours and sent to the laboratory to extract the excreted penicillin which was to be used again. There was striking improvement in the patient's condition by the fourth day. However, by the fifth day the supply of penicillin was exhausted. The patient's condition started to deteriorate and he died after a month of agonizing suffering.

Florey and his colleagues tried out the drug successfully in four other patients but were convinced that their laboratory in Oxford could not produce sufficient quantities of the drug for a proper clinical trial. British pharmaceutical companies when approached were too busy to attempt the manufacture of penicillin. Florey and Heatley in July 1941 therefore went to the US to enlist help in the production of the drug. Research on penicillin in the US was centred at the Northern Regional Research Laboratory at Illinois. Heatley worked with Andrew J. Moyer (1899-1959) at this laboratory for several weeks. Moyer extracted as much information from Heatley as possible but did not share his own findings. Moyer succeeded in increasing the yield of penicillin by 34 times. The US by now had entered the war, and both the Government and the US pharmaceutical companies showed top priority for the manufacture of the drug.

In 1942, Fleming asked for some penicillin to save a friend dying of acute infection. His friend who was given the drug recovered, and the report of this miraculous recovery appeared in the 'Times'. It was then that Almroth Wright wrote a letter ascribing the discovery of penicillin to his protégé—Fleming. The hall of fame now opened its doors to Alexander Fleming.

In 1943, British drug companies had also begun to produce penicillin in bulk. Florey went over to the war zone in North Africa and proved the successful use of the drug on battle wounds. The drug was also found extremely useful in the treatment of gonorrhea, a disease afflicting several soldiers in the war. By D-day 6 June 1944, penicillin was freely available to treat all allied servicemen. The Germans, Italians and Japanese never discovered the secret of penicillin; in a way the drug helped the Allies to win the war.

Fleming, Florey and Chain shared the Nobel prize in medicine in 1945 for the discovery and development of penicillin. Their achievement, however, went further for they clarified the principles underlying the discovery of all future antibiotics. In his acceptance speech, Florey enunciated these principles: the screening of organisms which produced a substance that was antibacterial, the extraction of this substance in a purified form; then testing the substance for toxicity, investigating its antibacterial properties in animal experiments and finally trying it out on humans. The screening of tens of thousands of organisms over the next 20 to 30 years, chiefly fungi, resulted in the discovery of a small number that produced a wide range of antibiotics active against numerous different infections. Penicillin is thus the wonder drug that ushered in an antibiotic revolution.

It is now over 65 years since penicillin was first used on the policeman Albert Alexander; we can therefore view this discovery in a better perspective. It was unquestionably an important discovery but it was not exactly a triumph of science in the true sense of the term. It was not a discovery through design, but a discovery through chance or accident. The unusual climatic conditions which led to Fleming's discovery of the antibacterial properties of the penicillium mould were fortuitous. Credit to Fleming that he did not throw away the Petri dish showing lysed bacteria around the penicillium mould as 'contaminated' and for having pursued investigations on the antibacterial effects of the mould. Then all was forgotten! Florey resuscitated what was till then a dead discovery and it was the world war that spurred him to investigate further. Had it not been for the war, Florey would almost certainly have never converted his laboratory to a manufacturing unit for penicillin and it is doubtful if the discovery of penicillin could have matured to benefit mankind.

The discovery of penicillin and of other antibiotics that followed this discovery aroused great euphoria among both doctors and patients. To rid the world of infection and infectious diseases was a thrilling prospect. Yet from today's vantage point, this did not quite materialize. Microbes, like man, evolve. When threatened with extinction they evolve so as to be resistant to antibiotics. Resistant organisms as for example the resistant staphylococcus and the resistant tubercle bacillus pose a great threat to humanity. Also, new infections caused by micro-organisms that were unrecognized earlier or that mutate to become virulent can cause fresh problems and pose fresh challenges to medicine and science. It is apparent that we live in an ecological balance with these microscopic creatures and that eliminating all micro-organisms in their entirety is not possible and perhaps not desirable. We shall continue to learn to cope with them just as much as they will adapt and continue to cope with us.

Finally we ask, why do a few micro-organisms produce chemical substances that destroy other bacteria? Selman Waksman, the discoverer of streptomycin for the treatment of tuberculosis, first postulated that these chemical substances or antibiotics protected the micro-organisms producing them from other bacteria. There are many reasons to believe that this indeed is not so. But then what purpose do they serve in nature? It is difficult to conceive that simple micro-organisms should produce complex chemical substances which play no role in their survival. This is a mystery that poses a challenge to science.

The second landmark discovery that I have chosen is the discovery of cortisone. The discovery of cortisone has been credited to Dr Philip Hench who in 1948 was the first to demonstrate its dramatic efficacy in rheumatoid arthritis. Dr Philip Hench was head of the Division of Medicine at the Mayo Clinic in Rochester, New York State. He was a large man with a wide cleft palate, so it was difficult to understand him at times when he spoke. An astute clinician, resolute and determined in his work and in what he set himself out to do, he rose in time to become a spellbinding lecturer, listened to with rapt attention by students and faculty members of the Mayo Clinic. It was indeed a magical moment in the history of medicine when he demonstrated the almost miraculous effect of cortisone to students and faculty in 1948.

The story of the discovery of cortisone begins 20 years prior, in 1928. A 65-year-old doctor suffering from rheumatoid arthritis was admitted to the Mayo Clinic under Dr Hench for an acute attack of jaundice which required both investigation and treatment. A chance discussion followed in which the doctor mentioned to Dr Hench that his joint pains, swelling and stiffness in his hands and feet had diminished markedly after the onset of jaundice and he could walk without pain for a mile. The jaundice had lasted for four weeks, but he was relatively free of pain, swelling and stiffness of joints for another seven months. This striking remission of rheumatoid arthritis obviously aroused a scientific curiosity in Dr Hench who in his manifold duties was also in charge of the rheumatology ward at the Mayo Clinic. Was this a mere coincidence? Or was there a cause and effect to this story? In a few years, he realized that the remission in rheumatoid disease that he had observed in his doctor patient was no coincidence, as he came across several other patients with jaundice who had the same experience. Dr Hench commented on his observation in a scientific paper published in the Proceedings of the Mayo Clinic in 1933. 'The therapeutic implications are obvious.

It would be gratifying to repeat nature's miracle to provide at will a similar beneficial effect by the use of some non-toxic accompaniment of jaundice.'

Hench concluded that there must be some agent that was responsible for the jaundice-induced remission of rheumatoid arthritis. He did not of course have the foggiest idea of what this 'agent' was, nor could he put his observation to practical use. He dubbed this unknown agent 'Substance X'. He logically questioned whether this chemical was in the bile of a jaundiced patient, or whether the jaundice stimulated the production of this chemical from somewhere outside the liver and biliary system. He tried to replicate nature's doing by feeding his patients with rheumatoid arthritis bile salts, liver extracts but without any effect. He even transfused his patients with blood taken from jaundiced patients but to no avail. He listed these failed attempts in an article published in the British Medical Journal in 1938, yet concluded his article thus—' It is important for us to identify nature's dramatic anecdotes....but the next step belongs to the future'.

Hench now made two further important observations. He noted that a remission in rheumatoid arthritis could also occur in pregnancy. He concluded from this observation that Substance X was not specifically related to jaundice, but was an unknown hormone whose concentration in blood increased with both jaundice and pregnancy. It not only produced a remission in rheumatoid arthritis but also in asthma, upper respiratory allergies, and at times in myasthenia gravis, a neurological disorder characterized by muscle fatiguability and weakness. Substance X thus in theory should not only relieve rheumatoid arthritis but other diverse unrelated illnesses as well. These were good observations, but that was as far as Hench could go. The identity of Substance X (later termed as cortisone) remained as nebulous, mysterious and undetermined as before. And indeed it would have remained so, had it not been for Professor Edward Kendall, Professor of Physiological Chemistry at the Mayo Clinic, who ultimately provided the answer to the identity of Substance X.

Kendall was indeed an excellent research scholar. As a young man of 28, he had isolated thyroxine (hormone secreted by the thyroid gland). Now as Professor of Physiological Chemistry he was interested in the hormonal secretion of the adrenal glands, (two glands sitting on top of the kidneys). The clinical condition produced by destruction of the adrenal glands (either from tuberculosis or atrophy) was known as Addison's disease following the classic description given by Dr Thomas Addison of Guy's Hospital, London, way back in 1855. This disease was characterized by fatiguability, extreme weakness, weight loss, anaemia, hypotension and a dark pigmentation of the skin and mucosa. It was fatal within six to twelve months. Patients with Addison's disease were treated by a compound made from adrenal glands of cats, but the natural identity of the hormone is secreted by the adrenals was unknown. In 1929, Kendall set out to determine the identity of these hormones. This was around the same time as Hench's discussion with his doctor patient on the remission of rheumatoid arthritis with jaundice and his thinking of a Substance X responsible for this remission. By 1932, Kendall together with other research scientists had isolated several chemical compounds from the adrenal glands which were known as compounds A, B, E, F.

Hench and Kendall working in the same institute became friends and exchanged ideas on their work. They wondered if Substance X could be either A, B, E or F. This, however, remained a mere conjecture for which there was absolutely no evidence. This was one reason why pharmaceutical companies did not show interest in manufacturing these compounds in sufficient quantities.

Then came the Second World War, which brought with it a dramatic change in the odyssey that led to the discovery of cortisone. In 1941, US intelligence agents reported that Nazi Germany was purchasing large quantities of adrenal glands from cattle in Argentina. There was a rumour that Luftwaffe pilots were injected with extracts of these adrenal glands following which they could fly unscathed at altitudes of 40,000 ft. The US Air force promptly started a research programme in all research institutes in the US and Canada that had worked on the adrenal glands. The rumour of Luftwaffe pilots flying at extraordinary high altitudes after being primed with adrenal cortex extracts was wrong, but the rumour had set in motion a strongly motivated research programme that ultimately bore fruit. It was however as late as 1948 that Dr Lewis Sarett working with Merck was able to synthesize a few grams of pure Compound E which was soon to be named cortisone.

We now go back to the rheumatology ward of Dr Philip Hench. A young woman of 29, Mrs Gardner was admitted under his care on 26 July 1948. She had severe rheumatoid arthritis and over a period of the next two months was hopelessly crippled, could walk with great difficulty and was for all purposes confined to a wheelchair. Hench spoke about this unfortunate patient to Kendall, who informed him that the pharmaceutical company Merck, had just succeeded in synthesizing a small quantity of Compound E, now called cortisone, secreted by the adrenal glands. Hench requested for the supply of this drug. The next day a small quantity of Compound E arrived in a package by airmail. Hench began with daily injections of 100 mg to Mrs Gardner. There was no change on the first day but two days later there was a dramatic improvement—her muscle stiffness had disappeared, she could get out of bed and could walk comfortably except for a slight limp. Four days later, her mobility was so miraculously improved that she could go shopping into town. For a patient who had been previously confined to a wheelchair, this seemed like a miraculous cure.

Dr Philip Hench treated a further 13 severely afflicted patients having rheumatoid arthritis with Compound E (cortisone)—again with dramatic results. He presented the results of this work to his fellow physicians at the Mayo Clinic at a meeting in April 1949. I quote the following lines from Albert Masel's book *The Hormone Quest*. 'The lights were turned down and a colour film began flickering on the screen. First came the 'before treatment' pictures in which patients struggled to take a few steps. Suddenly an electrifying gasp swept through the audience as the 'after treatment' scenes appeared and the doctors saw the very same patients jauntily climbing steps, swinging their arms and legs and even doing a little jig as if they had never been crippled at all. Even before the film ended, the watching physicians had filled the hall with wave after wave of resounding applause. When the lights went up and Dr Hench approached the lectern, he was greeted with a standing ovation.'

Following this 1949 clinical meeting wherein Hench demonstrated the miraculous effect of Compound E on rheumatoid arthritis, cortisone was presented as a genuine miracle cure. The following year Hench and Kendall were awarded the Nobel Prize. No Nobel Prize has been ever awarded so rapidly. In his acceptance speech, Hench donated a part of his prize money to Sister Pantaleon, the nun in charge of his rheumatology ward for several years, so that she could satisfy her wish to travel to Rome and meet the Pope.

Alas! Cortisone was not the miracle cure it was initially thought to be. As soon as the treatment stopped, the crippling features of rheumatoid arthritis returned with increased fury. What is more its prolonged use produced numerous side-effects—moon-face, obesity, increased blood sugar levels, hypertension, gastric ulcers which could perforate and bleed, osteoporotic fractures of bones, susceptibility to intercurrent infections. Hench soon became aware of the side-effects of cortisone; he was dejected and depressed for he soon realized that this drug was no miracle cure for rheumatoid arthritis. It was sad to have spent a lifetime in discovering a cure for an hitherto untreatable disease only to find that not only was the discovery not a cure but that it could cause dangerous side-effects. Cortisone today is used sparingly in rheumatoid disease and that too only under specific circumstances. Its reputation as a miracle cure in rheumatoid disease plummeted fast, but unwittingly and surprisingly it proved an excellent therapeutic tool for several other unrelated illnesses. Cortisone and its derivatives, often termed 'steroids', are today used in diseases involving several separate specialities—in gastroenterology, pulmonary medicine, nephrology, rheumatology, dermatology, ophthalmology. They are vitally useful in the management of acute anaphylaxis, in autoimmune disorders (classically in systemic lupus) as also to prevent rejection of organ transplants. The modus operandi of this drug in several diverse diseases is still not quite understood and technical details of research on this aspect of the drug would not interest the lay reader. It modulates the inflammatory process that accompanies several diseases to the patient's advantage. It generally does not cure, but when correctly used, relieves, alleviates or controls several disease processes.

When we look back in time at the story of cortisone it becomes apparent that the discovery was possible only because of a combination of fortunate circumstances. Hench's clinical acumen made him realize that the temporary remission of rheumatoid arthritis in patients with jaundice and in pregnancy was related to an unknown substance (Substance X). He had absolutely no clue what this substance was, though he did postulate that it could be a hormone. A lesser clinician perhaps may not have made this clinical observation and even if he had done so, would probably have ignored it or not followed it up. Hench however persisted in his search for Substance X with single-minded determination.

It was entirely fortuitous that around the same time Campbell working in the same institute was researching on the hormones secreted by the adrenal glands. At that point in time there was no clinical or experimental evidence to suggest that a hormone secreted by the adrenal gland would in fact be Substance X. Campbell was clever enough to isolate and synthesize very small quantities of compounds A, B, E, F from the adrenals but no pharmaceutical company would undertake manufacturing of these compounds because of a total lack of evidence that any one of these compounds could cause a remission in rheumatoid arthritis.

The exigencies imposed by the Second World War changed this scenario. The rumour that Luftwaffe pilots were given adrenocortical extracts to improve their flying performance led the US command to start and accelerate the research on adrenocortical hormones resulting in the availability of Compound E through Merck pharmaceuticals. These were all fortuitous circumstances. Had they been absent the discovery of cortisone may well have been delayed by several years.

Finally Compound E was tried on Mrs Gardner, perhaps as an intuitive thought. The reason for its use was not based on theory or experimental work. It is also worth knowing that when Hench used cortisone on Mrs Gardner, for some unknown reason he used a larger dose (100 mg) in relation to hormone requirement for a deficiency of this hormone. Had he used a smaller dose there probably would have not been any beneficial result and the discovery of cortisone might perhaps have been missed. Also the size of the crystals in the injectable preparations was exactly correct allowing quick absorption of the drug. Had they been larger, the absorption would have been delayed and the effect less marked.

Hench's determination paid off but as James Le Fanu writes, 'He got it right for the wrong reasons'. Cortisone today is far more useful for numerous other diseases than it is for rheumatoid arthritis.

The third landmark in modern medicine I shall now describe is the unravelling of the structure of deoxyribonucleic acid (DNA) by James Watson and Francis Crick in 1953. It constitutes the unmasking of the very structure of life, the biochemistry of existence and is perhaps the most momentous and important medical and scientific discovery of the twentieth century. This discovery I feel is on par with Harvey's discovery of circulation and of Pasteur's proven concept that diseases are not due to 'miasmas' floating in the air (as was once believed) but due to micro-organisms, and that a specific micro-organism was responsible for a specific disease. Interestingly enough, Watson and Crick were not doctors of medicine; they were physicists just as Pasteur was a chemist. The contribution of basic sciences to outstanding discoveries in medicine cannot be overemphasized. Most great discoveries have a backing of preparatory research done by earlier researchers. This preparatory research then becomes a prelude to the ultimate or final discovery. Earlier work on the unravelling of the structure of life, the biochemistry of existence was, however, meagre and it would be of interest to know what research on this subject preceded the final discovery of Watson and Crick.

In 1869, the Swiss scientist Friedrich Miescher discovered that an identical substance was present in the nucleus of every living cell. He called this nuclein, later changed to nucleic acid. At the beginning of the twentieth century biochemists had determined that the nucleic acid molecule contained five chemical bases—guanine (G), adenine (A), cytosine (C), thymine (T), and uracil (U). By the 1920s, two forms of nucleic acid were identified—DNA (deoxyribonucleic acid) and RNA (ribonucleic acid). The belief among many scientists was that the DNA structure was simple and repetitive and this could not transmit information. It was Edwin Schrodinger, a pioneer in quantum physics who disputed this view. In 1944, in a little book called *What is life?*, he described the unit responsible for heredity in purely molecular terms. He likened it to an 'aperiodic crystal', a structure obeying fundamental laws of physics but not repetitive, so that it was capable of holding a large amount of coded matter. It was this crucial description that sparked and attracted the attention of a number of physicists who till then had not researched on living matter. Maurice Wilkins, Francis Crick and James Watson took up the challenge to discover the exact biochemistry of existence. Let me briefly describe how this challenge was successfully met.

Maurice Wilkins was as assistant director in the Medical Research Council (MRC), Biophysics Unit, at King's College, London. He was given a pure sample of DNA and using a hurriedly assembled X-ray diffraction equipment, he obtained spotted patterns produced when DNA was pulled to form a thin fibre. The spotted pattern suggested a helix but he lacked the expertise to interpret this X-ray finding. This was provided by Rosalind Franklin, who having worked on the structure of coal, joined the team at King's College on the understanding that she would take over the study of DNA from Wilkins. Wilkins however continued, treated Franklin as a junior, causing bitterness and acrimony not conducive to successful research.

In 1949, Francis Crick, a 33-year-old physicist joined the MRC's unit at Cambridge University as a research student. He was joined two years later by James Watson, a brilliant 23-year-old American physicist, a famous child prodigy, who had entered Chicago University at the age of fifteen. Neither knew much biochemistry but both realized that no DNA research was possible without X-ray diffraction data. Crick knew that this research was also being carried out at King's College. Crick and Watson established a rapport with Wilkins of King's College, who discussed his work on the DNA with them. Watson and Crick built their first model of the DNA based on the theory by Linus Pauling that the structure comprised a triple helix. Wilkins brought Franklin to see this model and she showed that the idea of a triple helix was totally incompatible with her X-ray data. Disappointed, Watson and Crick stopped their research on DNA for nearly six months.

In January 1953, two events spurred the researchers on once again. Peter Pauling showed Watson a paper his famous father was about to publish regarding the structure of the DNA as a triple helix with phosphate backbones inside. Watson and Crick knew from their own previous mistake that this had to be wrong. It would take six weeks for Pauling's paper to be published—the two young researchers gave themselves this span of time to come up with the right answers. Fate was now kind to them. Wilkins gave Watson (without Franklin's permission) a print of one of Franklin's best X-ray photographs of the DNA. This print told Watson that the structure of the DNA was a double helix. They hurriedly began another model in which they placed the backbones on the inside with the bases sticking out. They realized their mistake when they compared this model to Franklin's X-ray print and changed their model so that the backbones were on the outside and the bases on the inside. The final model resembled a twisted ladder with the bases as the rungs. It took another week for them to assemble the bases in correct order. Watson and Crick completed the final correct model on 7 March 1953 and the results of their discovery were published in a short paper in Nature on 25 April 1953.

It is of interest that two teams were engaged in the same research—Maurice Wilkins, Rosalind Franklin at King's College, London and Francis Crick, James Watson at Cambridge. In a way, it was the bitterness, acrimony and the poor cooperation between Wilkins and Franklin that indirectly helped Watson and Crick to first solve the problem. Wilkins gave away extremely important information when he surreptitiously and without Franklin's consent gave Watson a print of one of Franklin's best photographs of the DNA. It was this print that made Watson conclude that the structure of DNA was a double helix and this set the Cambridge team on the road to success. It will remain a matter of conjecture as to the shape of events if Watson had not received this vital clue. Rosalind Franklin never realized how much Watson and Crick's discovery was due to her data, because she was unaware that they had seen an X-ray photograph of the DNA prior to the construction of the correct model. The vagaries of fate and fortune therefore played a significant role in Watson and Crick's success. In 1962, Watson, Crick and Wilkins were awarded the Nobel Prize for physiology and medicine. Rosalind Franklin surely deserved to share this prize but she had unfortunately died of cancer in 1958.

The biochemistry of life was solved and it was accepted that a complicated genetic code could be contained in the DNA. The field of genetics was now wide open. In the 1980s it became possible to chemically read the genetic code, to isolate genes and to duplicate (i.e. clone) them. Through the study of amniotic fluid (amniocentesis), it now became possible to screen a foetus *in utero* for genetic defects, so that a number of congenital defects could be diagnosed before birth. The isolation of a gene responsible for a particular disease either because it does not reproduce a specific gene product or produces an abnormal product holds great attraction both to the theory and practice of medicine. A revolution in gene discovery is currently afoot. The human genome project initiated in 1990 was completed by 2000, five years before its expected completion. Molecular biology, genetic medicine, advances in reproductive physiology form the frontiers of medicine today and will probably play an increasing role in the future. The foundation stone of future medicine may well be the unravelling of the basic structure of life—the DNA, 55 years ago.

Art and Medicine

Disease was the most basic ground
Of my creative urge and stress:
Creating, I could convalesce
Creating, I again grew sound.

—Heinrich Heine

This essay stems from an urge to explore the relationship between Art and Medicine. Medicine is in equal measure an art and a science and has close links with the humanities—with history, the visual arts, literature, poetry and music. The pursuit of the humanities is verily a study of Mankind but 'the best study of Mankind is Man'. Medicine is a never-ending quest of the study of Man—not just the working of the physical body, but of the mind, the relationship between man and his environment and of man as an integral part of nature. Both art and medicine reach out towards the same goal, though they may do so through different means and in different directions. There can be no art without artists and medicine cannot exist without physicians, and of what use are physicians, if there are no patients. The pursuit of art and the pursuit of medicine, like the pursuit of numerous other endeavours centres around man.

Medicine was born with the awakening of consciousness in man; art as related to medicine must have followed later, by depicting in art forms the methods of primitive caring and then of primitive healing. This relationship strengthened with the passage of time. Today, the most obvious relationship between visual art and medicine is the depiction of various deformities, defects and diseases in paintings. Defects such as blindness, cleft lip, and deformities such as dwarfism, achondroplasia have been brilliantly depicted by various artists. To give an example, the dwarf Maribarbola in Velasquez' famous painting 'Las Meninas' is beautifully portrayed; no textbook description could improve upon this masterly portrayal. Madness too, in all its forms has found frequent expression by artists through the ages.

More importantly, visual art provides a visual history of medicine and with it the visual history of civilization and of man from antiquity to modern times, embracing varying cultures and different societies in our world. It explores the march of medicine from ancient civilization to our present era, relating in pictorial form the tale of healers and would-be healers, their role and their relation to society. Visual art also explores the doctor-patient relationship, bringing out the empathy that needs to exist between the doctor and the patient as also the compassion, care and humanity that constitute the core of medicine. Two works of art illustrate this beautifully—the first, a painting by Sir Luke Fildes, titled 'The Doctor' and the other titled 'Science and Charity', painted by Pablo Picasso when he was just 15 years old. Another aspect of the relationship between art and medicine is the depiction of diagnostic techniques and modes of medical treatment in works of art. Paintings depicting the above relationship would fill more than one large volume. I shall rest content by choosing just a few examples of visual art with short descriptions beneath each.

The relationship between art and medicine is not just confined to the visual arts; it is also observed in literature and poetry. Authors and poets suffering from a particular disease, defect or deformity have either given brilliant descriptions in literature or verse of what they suffered from, or have depicted these ailments in their fictional characters. I shall illustrate this briefly later. But at this point I shall quote from the plays of the great bard William Shakespeare merely to show how he was acutely aware of death and disease in the society of his time.

There are well over 200 references in Shakespeare's plays to diseases of the body and mind. Numerous ailments including heart diseases, epilepsy, insanity, diseases of the eyes, wounds, haemorrhagic disorders, gynaecological disorders, syphilis, plague, rabies have been mentioned or briefly described. In his play *Othello*, the moor when convinced of Desdemona's guilt, gets an attack of epilepsy, which prompts Iago to say—

'This is his second fit; he had one yesterday.
The lethargy must have his quiet course,
If not, he foams at the mouth and by and by
Breaks out to savage madness.'

The bard also mentions many infectious diseases. In *King Henry V* there is a brief illusion to the illness of Falstaff, who is 'so shaken of a burning quotidian tertian that it is most lamentable to behold' . This description of intermittent fever with rigors suggests malaria or septic fever.

Then again palpitation or an acute awareness of the heart beat is beautifully versified in the *Winter's Tale*

'I have tremor cordis on me,—my heart dances'.

Perhaps we could read into the illness of Cardinal Beaufort in *King Henry VII*, a possible description of coronary thrombosis or a heart attack which was unheard of in the days of Shakespeare.

'That Cardinal Beaufort is at point of death;
For suddenly a grievous sickness took him
That makes him gasp and stare and catch the air'

Shakespeare's ideal of what a doctor should be is described in *All's Well that Ends Well*—

'One whose skill was almost as great as his honesty,
had it stretched so far would have made nature immortal
and death should have play for lack of work.'

Let me now explore the relationship between music and medicine. 'The heart that is not moved by music is fit for tyranny, stratagem and spoil.' Music to me and to many in this world is the greatest of all arts. Great music can induce a state of ecstatic joy, or lull one into a state of contemplative, detached serenity, or arouse passions that make the heart tremble with excitement. Great music in rare moments enables one to reach deep within one's buried psyche, and then transcend outwards, stretching out to infinity so as to commune with God. Music can be the most emotive of all the arts, followed by poetry and then perhaps by literature and the visual arts. The written word either in prose or verse, the visual impact of a great painting or sculpture can lead to thoughts and impressions that have a neurophysiological basis. We hear music with our ears, but the mechanism of its emotive response, or of the overall musical experience is a mystery that has remained unsolved. To quote Claude Levi Strauss,

'Since music is the only language with the contrary attributes of being at once intelligible and untranslatable, the musical creator is a being comparable to gods, and music itself the supreme mystery of the science of man.'

'Music hath the power to soothe the savage breast.' It also has the power to assuage suffering, to confer calm and peace to a troubled mind. Studies have shown that music is helpful to patients; it induces a state of relaxation, can reduce blood pressure, heart rate, stress hormones, pain and the need for pain medication. It can lift depression, eliminate fear, induce positive thoughts, enabling the patient to fight disease successfully. It is being increasingly used in cancer patients, where a positive approach induced by listening daily to music, or performing it singly or in a group goes a long way in achieving a better outcome. Appropriate music must needs be used for this purpose, for just as some music can soothe and calm, other music can excite, and produce undesirable physiological changes within the body. I have used music therapy in the hospital and have advised music therapy in selected patients in my consulting practice. There are some works of music which are indeed particularly effective. When heard in a quiet room, more so in the stillness of the night, when most pain is felt more deeply, and when troubles may turn to nightmares, these works help to relieve suffering and calm the mind.

Let me give just a few of the many examples of these musical works. I frequently recommend the music of Mozart, in particular his clarinet concerto, some of his sonatas for the violin and piano, the Andante of his piano concerto in G major, and much of his chamber music. Bach is equally wonderful to listen to, particularly for an individual with a trained musical ear. His music weaves a spiritual web and produces a trance-like effect which assuages physical or mental suffering. Beethoven's music, his sonatas, his violin concerto, particularly the second movement, Chopin's nocturnes can act likewise. However, it is not just Western classical music that exerts this effect. It can be any music from any part of the world, as long as it soothes and has a special appeal for the listener. It is important to ask the patient to concentrate deeply on the music that he hears, to listen to every note, to shut out noises from the mind, to banish any outside thought that may arise in the mind's eye as promptly as possible. The more intense the focus on the music the greater its effect. For those who appreciate Indian music, I recommend the flute of Pandit Hariprasad Chaurasia, soothing ragas played on the sitar by Pandit Ravi Shankar, and the melodious shehnai of Ustad Bismillah Khan. I have found music therapy particularly useful in postoperative patients to counter pain and depression, or to lift the mental trauma, fear, fright in patients with cancer, either following a diagnosis or following surgery and chemotherapy.

Music therapy is not new. It was used in the Second World War to help soldiers convalesce from wounds, trauma and surgery. The art and science of Ayurveda was familiar with music as a form of treatment. An ancient Indian study known as Nada Yoga acknowledges the effect of different Ragas (sounds and vibrations) on the mind and body. This has come down to us as the Raga Chikitsa, which is really music therapy. According to the Raga Chikitsa, different ragas are prescribed for different ailments. For example, the Todi Raga is believed to relieve hypertension, Marwa Raga to relieve fever.

How does music therapy help to alleviate pain and suffering? To the extent that music heals, how does it heal? Music obviously acts on the mind-body complex, though the exact physiological pathways remain obscure. Recent published research by Dr Conrad and his colleagues suggest that the physiological response of critically ill patients exposed to the soothing music of Mozart was characterized by an unexpected jump in the pituitary growth hormone, which is known to be crucial in healing. Earlier reports suggest that listening to Mozart's music can lead to an increased activation of brain regions that are not directly involved in the process of listening. Music may thus act through the neuroendocrine system which is in a way, a neuronal orchestra conductor directing the body's immune system. Music perhaps stimulates this conductor to get the healing process started. Dr Conrad plans further studies on how music can improve a surgeon's performance. Let me quote Dr Conrad on this subject—'If I don't play music for a couple of days, I cannot feel things as well in surgery. My hands are not as tender with the tissue. They are not as sensitive to the feedback that the tissue gives you.'

Professor Michael Schulte Markwood, Head of Child Psychology at Hamburg's University Hospital in Germany has used music therapy on unruly children. He noted the calming effect of the therapy together with an improvement in their physical coordination and cognitive skills. He also maintains that experimental work suggests that unborn babies in the womb appear to relax in response to certain music, and amazingly seem to recognize this music after birth.

I feel music benefits man, it pleases, elevates and at times ennobles the human spirit. It is increasingly evident that its effect on the mind-body complex adds to the healing power of medicine. I am inclined to agree with Joseph Addison—

'Music the greatest good that mortals know
And all of heaven we have below'.

There is one special important aspect of the art-medicine relationship which has not yet been touched upon. Does disease, mental illness, physical deformity or defect influence great art or more importantly the creativity of an artist? I refer to truly great art. I speak of art which is arresting, often stupefying; art which arouses a strong emotive response, 'art that has the wings of a bird' and transports one to an other-worldly, soul-shattering experience.

The question asked above arouses a fair degree of controversy. There are some who believe that illness and suffering in great artists are incidental factors in life and to ascribe these, as a cause of creativity is unjustified. Yet there are others who like me believe that suffering in any form does affect creativity in an artist. More often than not suffering sparks creativity, lights a fire,—and great art is born.

Many artists in different fields of art have indeed testified to this effect. Before I quote their views I feel it is important to ask another relevant question. What is the source of great art, what is its genesis? An answer to this question would perhaps help us to understand how and why physical or emotional torment can influence it.

Great art cannot be created in a vacuum; it cannot arise from nothing; nor can it arise solely as an invention or a figment of imagination. Great art springs from the experiences that the world and life offer or force upon an artist. It is this collective experience, often buried deep within the unconscious, that becomes the source of artistic creation. But we all have experience; each one also has his or her own share of suffering, and yet we are not great artists! Then, where lies the difference? It lies in the ability of the artist to see the world differently, perhaps to see the world as the world is not; to feel intensely, to imagine vividly. It also lies in being able to delve deep into the regions of the unconscious psyche, draw forth hidden emotions from buried experiences to a conscious level, and then transmute these into great art. It is feeling rather than intellect that enables an artist to transform experience, transcend reality, so as to reach a point beyond it. What enables a great artist to do so? This is a question that admits no answer. It is a gift either inborn or acquired, that enables him to do so; an attempt to describe the genesis of this gift would be an exercise in futility. At times this gift amounts to real genius, as in the case of Wolfgang Amadeus Mozart, who started composing at the age of six, when 'experience', overt or hidden hardly mattered.

The observations and remarks made above apply equally to music and abstract art. Mahler, the great Austrian composer has stressed the role of experience in musical composition. I quote from Alma Mahler's book *Gustav Mahler, Memories and Letters*—'Creative art and actual experience are one and the same.' He then goes on to say —'However a bit of mystery always remains for the creator.' The 'mystery' is transforming his 'experience' into great music.

Mondrian, an exponent of abstract art believes the same—'all that the nonfigurative artist receives from outside is not only useful but indispensable, because it arouses in him the desire to create that which he only vaguely feels and which he could never represent in a true manner without the contact with visible reality and with the world which surrounds him'.

I will now quote the views of just a few of the many in the art world, who believed that suffering and pain, either from disease, defect or disability enhanced their creativity.

Let me start with Thomas Mann who wrote, 'Great artists are great invalids'.

T. S. Eliot, one of the pioneers of modern English poetry has written an introduction to Pascal's *Pensées*. He writes in this introduction—'ill health not only favoured religious illumination, but also artistic and literary composition.' Nietzsche, the pioneer of modern philosophy was a tortured soul—a physical and emotional wreck both from disease and the vicissitudes of life. He was tormented with physical pain and from the numerous ailments that afflicted him. Yet he writes, 'I have never felt happier with myself than in the sickest periods of my life'. He believed that suffering spurred his creativity.

Emily Dickinson when threatened with blindness, versified thus—

'My loss, by sickness—was it loss? or ethereal gain
One earns by measuring the grave –
Then—measuring the sun.'

Deformity or defects have also sparked creativity in artists. Lord George Gordon Byron, a great poet who was plagued by constant pain in his club foot wrote—'An addiction to poetry is very generally the result of an uneasy mind in an uneasy body'.

It thus seems that not uncommonly a great artist is an unhappy being, whose heart torn asunder by grief and suffering, inspires him at times to ecstatic heights. He plucks at his anguished heart strings and the sound of sweet music fills the world.

I would now like to consider the relation between just a few important specific ailments and art and creativity. I shall first consider mental illness, then go on to the effect of deformities, to loss of sight and hearing and finally the relation of tuberculosis to creative art.

Genius is oft considered to be half mad. Many artists though outwardly normal have odd psychiatric features that perhaps contribute to their art. Some have hovered close to the thin line separating sanity from insanity, only to cross this line back and forth or forever. Genius is always treated with far greater latitude and consideration, so that what would be considered as a morbid psychiatric trait in an ordinary individual is condoned as an oddity or eccentricity in the genius. However, serious mental illnesses often have a marked effect on art, artistic talent and artistic creativity. For example, art works of the insane give an insight into the nature of the mental disorders they suffer from and may help both in diagnosis and in approach to management. Again, patients who are in the throes of a depressive illness or who are deeply melancholic, are prisoners imprisoned within the confines of their solitary selves, divorced from reality and the outside world. There is an urge to establish contact with reality and reach out to their fellow-men, but they are unable to break the shackles confining them. If such individuals could be induced to paint, write, versify, play or compose music, they would experience great relief, a feeling of deliverance from a veritable hell. Art in such instances has significant therapeutic value, a cathartic effect, as it replaces suffering with creativity. Finally in some great artists, madness or near madness is a spur to artistic creativity. Madness then perhaps acts by liberating thoughts from narrow confines to a new blazing vista, so that one so stricken flies on wings of fancy and fantasy to Olympian heights.

'Men have called me mad; but the question is not yet settled, whether madness is or is not the loftiest intelligence—whether much that is glorious—whether all that is profound—does not spring from disease of thought—from moods of mind exalted at the expense of the general intellect.'—*Edgar Allan Poe*

A number of great artists have been frankly schizophrenic or bordered on paranoia. Philip Sandblom in his excellent book *Creativity and Disease* cites several such examples, of which the most striking is Freidrich Holderlin, who following a broken romantic liaison, developed catatonic schizophrenia at the young age of thirty-two. His insanity changed his writing, and was reflected in his poetry. There was a connection between his art and progressive insanity. It is astonishing that his creative force scintillated both with regard to originality and linguistic strength as his madness worsened.

The influence of insanity on art can also be seen in the work of Edward Munch, the great Norwegian painter. His art was influenced by extreme anxiety and paranoia. The world famous painting titled 'The Shriek' shows a tormented figure emitting a heart-rending, horrific 'primal scream'. The painting trembles with agitation and anxiety, heightened by the artist's delirious brush-strokes, a reflection of his own despair and torment. This is what the artist had to say, ' I was ill and tired—I stood there, watching the fjord. I felt as if a shriek went through nature.'

A number of artists have suffered from a manic depressive state. Their work either reflects their agitation amounting at times to near mania or their underlying depression and melancholy, or both. Philip Sandblom includes Lord Byron, Virginia Woolf, Sylvia Plath and Kay Jamison among those so afflicted. Lord Byron poured his torment and misery in some of his letters, while Virginia Woolf transferred her agitation and depression into her fictional characters.

In *Mrs. Dalloway*, one of her famous novels, she brings out the consciousness of tyranny over the individual, while the novel *To The Lighthouse* focuses on the self-doubt and tension that eat into the individual. She herself was tortured by these very emotions, and poured out her torment with artistic creativity into her fictional works. Leonard Woolf, her husband, published extracts from his wife's diary after her death concerning her work. They reveal intense excitement during composition, and depression, exhaustion and a sense of failure when her results fell short of her aims. She committed suicide during one of her fits of depression.

Sylvia Plath, an American poet was also manic depressive. She said 'I only write because there is a voice within me that will not be still'. She wrote with a tragic foreboding that was fulfilled when she killed herself.

Perhaps the best description of a manic depressive state that I have read is by Dr. Kay Jamison in her autobiography titled *An Unquiet Mind*. Jamison besides being manic depressive herself was also a psychiatrist. She therefore had a real insight into the tragedy she endured, so that her description of this dreadful mental state is both poetic and frightful. She states that her two striking examples of mania were herself and Lord Byron.

The creative artist struck with a manic depressive disorder oft delights in the manic phase. Let me quote from Jamison's autobiography, 'When you are high it is tremendous. The idea and feelings are fast and frequent like shooting stars—I have been aware of finding new corners in my mind and heart. Some of these corners were incredible and beautiful and took my breath away'. This shows a beautiful insight into the new vistas of light and beauty that have sparked creativity to greater heights in some artists afflicted with a manic or near manic state. Amazingly in her case, this heightened awareness and increased originality also helped her in her scientific pursuits. She mentions—' having fire in one's blood—is not without its benefit to the walls of academic medicine'.

Of course, when the manic state is severe, creativity is disjointed, uncontrolled and therefore shows a decline. This is because the flow of ideas, the euphoria, and excitement becomes chaotic. Confusion overcomes clarity.

Depression often follows mania and with it comes the overwhelming urge to suicide. Jamison eventually consented to treatment with lithium. This led to a bitter-sweet exchange of a comfortable and settled existence for a troubled but intensely lived past. One senses a nostalgia for her lost mania.

Philip Sandblom writes of another American poet, Edna St. Vincent Millay, who alternated between the darkness of depression and the overwhelming light and euphoria of mania. She described her feeling of depression, and the lifting of this 'darkness' in beautiful verse.

'How can I bear, buried here
While overhead the sky grows clear'.

Then again,

'All at once the heavy night
Fell from my eyes and I could see—
A drenched and dripping apple tree.'

And now perhaps the euphoria of early mania, or was it just an expression of irrepressible relief!

'I raised my quivering arms on high,
I laughed and laughed into the sky.'

Epilepsy has afflicted great minds—Caesar and Napoleon to name two great military geniuses; Petrarch, Pascal, Byron, Flaubert and Dostoevsky to name creative artists in the field of literature, philosophy and poetry. The disease did in no way blunt the creativity of these great minds. Is there an association between genius and epilepsy? Not really so—except perhaps in Dostoevsky. He described his pre-epilepsy aura as one of ecstatic transcendental beauty. Let me quote this description.

'The sensation of life, of being multiplied tenfold at that moment; all passion, all doubts, all unrests were resolved as in a higher peace; then a peace full of dear harmonious joy of hope. And then a scene suddenly as if something were opening up in the soul; an indescribable, an unknown light radiated, by which the ultimate essence of things were made visible and recognizable—this feeling is so strong and sweet that for a few seconds of this enjoyment one would readily exchange ten years of one's life, perhaps even one's whole life.'

The post-epileptic state in Dostoevsky aroused opposite feelings; it was associated with a sense of guilt, a despondency that crippled his work for a time. Dostoevsky's creative mind transferred the feelings he experienced both during his aura and his post-epileptic state into his literary works. His beautiful pre-seizure experiences help to mould the character of Prince Myshkin in his novel *The Idiot*, while the post-seizure feelings of guilt and shame are transferred to one of his characters in the *Brothers Karamazov*. Dostoevsky welcomes his disease and indirectly links his great creativity to its influence, when he says, 'it is a glorious heavenly merging with the highest synthesis of life.'

Tennyson was another great literary artist who during his walks would work himself up into 'walking trances' by continuously repeating his own name. He termed these trances, 'beneficial mystic visions'. They may well have been episodes of a temporal lobe epilepsy. The trance was often associated with a surge of poetic imagination, excitement and beauty, a mystic experience that fuelled his creativity.

Perhaps the most classic example of the influence of manic-depressive psychosis (and epilepsy) on creative art is observed in the work of the great painter Vincent Van Gogh in his last and most creative years. His artistic powers were liberated and found free abandon during his manic phase. Perhaps this mental state was further aggravated or even precipitated by his consumption of absinthe and alcohol. He suffered delirious phases, during one of which he cut off the lobe of his ear and presented it to a prostitute. He painted furiously, continuously, brilliantly during this period of his life. His paintings reveal the torment, anxiety and delirium within the mind. 'My brushes run as fast beneath my fingers as the bow over a violin.' The colour yellow dominated his paintings; the brush strokes were furious as if laid on in an uncontrolled delirious frenzy; flames of colour leap out of his canvas, perhaps mirroring the flames that were consuming his mind.

What must have caused and precipitated this dreadful mental crisis in this great artist? Perhaps it was the trials and tribulations of his early life as a struggling artist when he felt rejected and depressed, coupled with the fallout with the artist Paul Gauguin with whom he was eager to form a working artistic relationship. Perhaps it was the lack of recognition, the inner urge to be accepted, to succeed, the agony of failure which helped light the fire within his brain, which set it ablaze, enabling him to create works of rare brilliance, passion and beauty.

One great composer who composed with greater ease, fluency and creativity during the manic phase of a manic-depressive state was Robert Schumann. His obsessional phobias and mood swings started from his early twenties but in his later years he also showed a paranoid psychotic behaviour. He sometimes heard inner voices which urged him to compose. 'Music was with him all the time'; to use Berlioz's phrase, 'he was a man haunted by genius'. Yet some of his best works were produced during moods of extreme elation, amounting to mania. The fantasy in C Major was thus composed in just five days and his violin concerto in two weeks. The music composed during his very excitable phase appears at times agitated and discordant. The notation of extra-rapid tempi in these compositions may well reflect the rapidity of thoughts and ideas that must have flitted through his mind in his near manic state.

In his later years he developed features of a paranoid psychosis; he had auditory hallucinations of a musical note being played in his head, of hearing angels singing a beautiful melody which he attempted to write down. With increasing madness his artistry ran aground and was soon extinguished. He attempted suicide by throwing himself into the waters of the Rhine and was ultimately isolated in a mental asylum where he starved himself to death.

Modern philosophy started with Friedrich Nietzsche. His life was a saga of physical suffering and emotional torment. He contracted syphilis as a student and suffered from it in his later life. In fact the sheer exuberance of his writing, his philosophic, poetic, well-nigh Messianic outpourings to the world may at least partly have been conditioned by a form of syphilitic involvement of the brain, termed general paralysis of the insane.

In 1882–3, Nietzsche fell into a state of utter despondency and depression after a humiliating end to a brief affair with his mistress Lou Salome. In fact he became mentally unbalanced, living in utter solitude. Intellectually, emotionally, physically, he was all but exhausted. Yet in this state of crisis, perhaps because of it, his creativity began to stir anew; ideas, thoughts came flashing unasked for into his mind, and there burst forth from within him an outpouring of great philosophy and poetry—*Thus Spoke Zarathustra*. I have never read a better or more vivid account of what 'creativity' means to an artistic genius than the description given by Nietzsche of his experience during the writing of this great work. I quote,

'One hears, one does not seek; one takes, one does not ask who gives; a thought flashes up like lightning with necessity unfalteringly formed—I have never had any choice. An ecstasy, whose tremendous tension, sometimes discharges itself into a flood of tears...'

Before this great work, Nietzsche had preached a nihilistic philosophy. Now he had a positive message, a meaning to man's existence in the world. 'I teach you the superman. Man is something that should be overcome.'

'All Gods are dead, now we want the superman to live—let this be our last will, one day at the great noontide!'

Also,

'Sing and bubble over O Zarathustra, heal your soul with new songs, so that you may hear your great destiny—behold, you are the teacher of eternal recurrence'.

Finally,

'O Man! Attend!
What does deep midnight voice contend? '
'I slept my sleep,
The world is deep,
Deeper than day can comprehend,
Deep is its woe,
Joy—deeper than heart's agony:
Woe says : Fade! Go!
But all joy wants eternity,
Wants deep, deep eternity!'

Beautiful philosophy wrapped in beautiful poetry!

Thus Spoke Zarathustra is a work of genius; genius sparked by a state of near madness and physical suffering. Its counterpart in music, bearing the same name is the beautiful tone poem by Richard Strauss.

Mental ill-health is not just confined to the extreme forms of depressive manic psychosis and paranoid schizophrenia or to a mental state bordering on these two psychotic disorders. The milder forms of mental ill-health are characterized by severe unnatural anxiety, leading to anxiety states, panic attacks and to a neurotic disposition, termed pyschoneurosis. Marcel Proust was the famous French author whose neurotic disposition helped shape one of the great novels of the twentieth century *–A la recherche du temps perdu* (In search of lost time). This is a story of Proust's life, an autobiography told as an allegorical search for truth, in which Proust recalls experiences of the past in an attempt to recapture time lost. Proust was a sickly child with allergic asthma. His father was a doctor and he grew up at home in an atmosphere that induced an unnatural attention and preoccupation with bodily symptoms and disease, both with regard to himself and to others. After the death of his mother to whom he was closely attached, his psychoneurosis worsened. He shut himself in a bedroom which was sealed to exclude dust and pollen and lined with cork to shut off noise. The psychosomatic nature of his asthma was revealed, when in spite of these precautions, the mere picture of a rose on the wallpaper of his room triggered a severe asthmatic attack.

Proust became a recluse in the confines of his bedroom, but with a fevered, fervid imagination, fuelled by his neurotic disposition, he projected his own self as author, narrator and into the characters of this masterly work. To quote his own words—'Everything great in the world is created by neurotics.'

I now wish to give a few examples of how deformities and defects can influence both art and artistic creativity. Let me quote Francis Bacon—'Whosoever had anything fixed in his person that doth induce contempt, hath also perpetual spur in himself to rescue and deliver himself from scorn; therefore all deformed persons are extreme bold.'

Lord Byron suffered from a club foot, a congenital deformity which in his own words 'was the curse of his life'. He was ultra-sensitive about this deformity and any allusion to it triggered a terrific rage. His noble ancestry, his handsome debonair face, and the physical and mental trauma produced by his deformity combined perhaps to shape his arrogance, his scorn for some of his contemporary poets and above all for his great poetic genius. The role played by his deformity in spurring him to great heights is manifest in his own poetic words.

'Deformity is daring,
It is the essence to overtake mankind
By heart and soul and make itself the equal,
Ay, the superior of the rest. There is
A spur in its halt movements to become
All that the others cannot, in such things
As still are free to both, to compensate
For stepdame Nature's avarice at first!'

Byron further wrote these prophetic words,

'There is that within me which shall tire Torture and Time,
And breathe when I expire.'

Another good example of how deformity could have influenced creativity is exemplified by the great French artist Toulouse Lautrec. He like Byron was of noble ancestry but was grossly deformed—far more than Byron. He had very short legs and a deformed head. The emotional trauma, leave aside the physical discomfort, drove him to reject the world, in particular members of his class. He decided to paint, drink and live a promiscuous life in the brothels of Paris. Perhaps neither his appearance nor social class mattered in the brothels he visited; perhaps his attitude was a show of defiance, a rebellion against his physical deformity. His artistic creativity blossomed and flourished; his style was distinctive; he immortalized in his art the denizens of the brothels, and the nightlife of Paris. He ranks as one of the great painters of the nineteenth century.

The musical virtuoso Nicolo Paganini could well have in part owed his great technical skills and virtuosity as a violinist to a congenital physical affliction. In his youth he led a life of unashamed debauchery. The infirmities of his later years may well have been related to dissipated youth. He suffered horrendously through the greater part of his musical career. He was seized with attacks of abdominal pain, had laryngeal disease, was edentulous in his lower jaw and subsisted on a semi-liquid diet, together with numerous medications. He could have also suffered from tuberculosis and syphilis, though there is no definite evidence that this was indeed so. Cadaveric and demoniac in appearance, yet the most brilliant violinist that ever lived, it was as if the devil had taken upon himself to show what the violin was capable of.

Was this incredible technique and virtuosity related to an unusual bodily habitus? His left shoulder was higher than the right, probably because of continuous practice on the violin. He was known to rapidly initiate unusual movements of the wrist and fingers of the left hand. He was capable of hyperextension of the thumb, lateral movements of the distal phalanges and could hyperextend his reach on the violin so as to play in three positions without shifting his hold on the violin. Almost certainly (yet there is no way of proving this), the unusual dexterity and elasticity of the left hand was possible because of a congenital genetic defect termed the Ehlers Danlos Syndrome (where the typical feature is a marked increase in elasticity and in range of movements resulting in double-jointedness).

Thus the greatest violin virtuoso that ever lived probably owed at least a part of his virtuosity to a congenital defect. Paganini's musicianship of course could never have been possible had he lacked the basic musical genius and creativity which he expressed through the violin.

Impaired vision can affect both art and creativity in art. A classic example is that of Claude Monet, perhaps the greatest impressionist artist of his time. He developed senile cataracts in his later years and this had a profound influence on his art. Monet loved to paint the same subject at different times of the day, as the play of light produced different coloured impressions in his mind's eye. Colours thus appeared bright, vibrant in the day, somber and dark at dusk. Monet rendered these impressions with supreme artistry, delicacy and harmony. Developing cataracts blurred his vision—'I see everything in fog.' Forms took on a vague shape and his sense of colour changed. He painted more in red as the cataract filtered out most of the other colours. He was displeased with his art, though art critics felt that Monet was now breaking new grounds and opening new vistas in his work. He however knew better, recognized that his paintings were not as good as they used to be and destroyed several of his panels.

Monet had his cataracts removed, and now the colours of objects in nature seemed more exaggerated; he saw more 'blue' and when he expressed this impression on canvas he remained even more dissatisfied. Eventually, Monet's colour vision improved with the help of tinted glasses. He was overjoyed and started painting with great passion and completed his classic paintings of 'water lilies' floating on the surface of a shimmering sheet of water, reflecting the sky—all bathed in a wondrous, changing light.

Two great blind poets esteemed for the beauty of their work were Homer and Milton. Homer of ancient Greece, Greece of the heroic age, composed the *Odyssey*, a classic of Greek literature and poetry.

John Milton was a poet-prophet who like Homer was blind. Yet no English poet since Shakespeare has ever approached his eminence. Milton had the passion, intensity and drive that rivalled Dante. He was totally blind in his forties. His genius was at its peak in his later years and he composed his greatest verse *Paradise Lost and Paradise Regained* during and after his late fifties when he had been totally blind for several years. To most, blindness is a curse. Here was one great bard who was not only reconciled to this dreadful loss ('I say again that I have lost no more than the most inconsequential skin of things'), but sublimated this loss into experiencing an internal light, enabling him to write some of the most memorable and heroic lines in English poetry. Was not this dreadful infirmity the spur to the flowering of his creative genius, the 'light' that though extinguished 'without' shone strongly 'within'? Coupled with his blindness was the physical and emotional trauma caused by his imprisonment for his republican views and for defending the regicide of Charles I. He was already blind for seven years when he was imprisoned and had to endure the strong possibility of a dreadful public execution— hanging, being cut down when alive, having one's entrails ripped from the body and only then beheaded! His suffering unquestionably shaped his passions, which he poured out into immortal verse.

I quote from one of his lovely sonnets, showing not only his reconciliation to his dreadful loss, but also the triumph of his spirit over adversity.

'When I consider how my light is spent,
Ere half my days in this dark world and wide,
And that one talent which is death to hide
Lodged with me useless, though my soul more bent
To serve herewith my Maker, and present
My true account, lest He returning chide;
'Doth God exact day-labour, light denied?'
I fondly ask. But Patience, to prevent
That murmur, soon replies, 'God doth not need
Either man's work or His own gifts. Who best
Bear His mild yoke, they serve Him best. His state
Is kingly: thousands at His bidding speed,
And post o'er land and ocean without rest;
They also serve who only stand and wait.'

Let me quote just once more a verse from his poem, *Samson Agonistes*

'But he, though blind of sight,
Despised and thought extinguished quite,
With inward eyes illuminated,
His fiery virtue roused
From under ashes into sudden flame'.

For a creative artist, impaired hearing progressing to total deafness, is almost as great a cross to bear as impairment and final loss of vision. Perhaps total deafness is even worse, except of course when total blindness makes creation of visual art impossible. Deafness isolates the artist so that he loses contact with the outside world. He lives in deathly silence, in a silent world, imprisoned within himself. He resents this affliction, withdraws and becomes a social recluse. This is bound to affect the artist's psyche, which in turn will affect his creativity.

Francisco Goya, the great Spanish painter and Ludwig Van Beethoven, the great German composer were afflicted by deafness. Goya at the age of 47 was struck by an acute illness which left him paralyzed and blind for a short time and deaf for the rest of his life. The nature of this illness is obscure; it could have been due to an acute viral infection, though there is however a belief that it could have been caused by lead intoxication, leading to lead encephalopathy. This is because Goya's method of painting consisted of the extravagant application of colour to his canvas, with whatever was at hand, entailing perhaps a significant exposure to lead. Before this catastrophe, he was happy and cheerful; his early paintings reflected both in form and colour, the radiance, brightness and good cheer of his personality. However, after recovering from his illness, he gave vent to his despair, anger and frustration, using the most horrible subjects as his themes, as if he was exorcizing his torment and suffering on the canvas. His creative genius changed directions from the pleasant to the grotesque and ugly.

The greatest example of a creative genius struggling to cope with progressive deafness is Beethoven. He was struck by this dreadful disability in his twenties, at an age when his musical genius was just beginning to unfold, both as a composer and as a virtuoso performer. His impaired hearing inexorably progressed to total deafness when he was in his forties. To a composer and a virtuoso performer this was the unkindest and cruellest cut of all. He also suffered from respiratory illness, from pancreatitis and liver cirrhosis in his later years, brought on by immoderate consumption of alcohol. But it was the curse of deafness which at first seemed to overwhelm and frustrate him. However, in course of time not only did he learn to cope with this affliction, but perhaps because of it, and the agony he underwent, he poured forth sublime music which had the rare power to ennoble the human spirit. His Eroica symphony evokes the struggle and triumph of man against tyranny and oppression, a theme dominant during the French Revolution and in Napoleonic Europe. This symphony was dedicated to his then hero, Napoleon. Beethoven however tore it up when Napoleon crowned himself as the Emperor of France.

It is difficult for many people to reconcile the greatness, richness and beauty of his music with what they know of its creator. When progressive deafness made him aware that he would soon be imprisoned forever in a silent world, when he realized that he could no longer hear the sound of music which he loved, and for which he felt he was created, he was devastated. He became a dishevelled misanthropic man, irascible, with an explosive temper, a recluse who shunned the company of his fellow-men. He poured out his agony and frustration in the Heiligenstadt testament of 1802. This testament is dedicated to his two brothers and is perhaps the most touching of his letters, enabling all to realize the torment that shaped his external appearance and manner. Let me quote from this testament written when he was 32 years old and when the sceptre of increasing deafness was upon him. He contemplated suicide but decided that his art dictated that he struggle and live.

'For the last six years I have been afflicted with an incurable complaint which has been made worse by incompetent doctors....

Alas! How could I refer to the impairing of a sense which in me should be more perfectly developed than in other people, a sense which at one time I possessed in great perfection—joyfully I go to meet death—should it come before I have had an opportunity of developing all my artistic gifts, then in spite of my hard fate it would still come too soon—Farewell and when I am dead do not wholly forget me.'

Beethoven counselled 'patience' to himself when he realized that he was getting progressively deaf. Patience to come to terms with his affliction. Let me quote once again from his testament. 'Patience, they say, is what I must now choose for my guide, and I have done so—I hope my determination will remain firm to endure until it pleases the inexorable Parcae to cut the thread. Perhaps I shall get better, perhaps not; at any rate I am resigned.'

Unfortunately he did not get better; his deafness grew progressively worse and he was stone deaf in his forties. His total deafness isolated him from the world; he now lived only to compose, to create, and this he did to the great benefit and joy of posterity. His creative genius was like an indomitable force that sprang from deep within and though unable to hear the sound of his music, he felt it within the very depths of his being. The sadness of his plight was worsened by the fact that his deafness seemed to have no cause and no cure. For that matter, in spite of repeated autopsies done in later years, the aetiology of his deafness even today is obscure.

His compositions now alternated between tumultuous passion and defiance, contrasting with resignation and calm as after a storm. Thus the Appassionata Sonata expresses the torment and tumult within a troubled mind. The Pastorale Symphony radiates an ethereal grace, and a beautiful serenity, as if he was reconciled to his fate and had surmounted his distress. His fifth symphony is 'Fate knocking at the door'. It is tragic to start with; the final movement however is almost joyous; again a triumph over fate and the sadness he harboured, as if he was now smiling at the world.

Beethoven's final works, the Ninth symphony as also the Mass in D showed him at the height of his powers as a composer. The music soars upwards, ennobles, reaching celestial heights. His life and creativity in music mirror our human condition, man's struggle and existence against the unpredictable vagaries of Fate. Let me quote his views on the creativity of his art—'The true artist has no pride; unhappily he realizes that art has no limitation. He feels darkly how far he is away from the goal and while perhaps he is admired by others, he has not reached the point where the better genius will shine before him like the distant sun.'

Beethoven died on 26 March 1827 at 6 pm amidst a dreadful thunderstorm. Perhaps the gods wished to welcome him with great éclat. He received extreme unction two days earlier and then wrote in his conversation book, 'Plaudite, amici, comedia finita est' (Applaud my friends, the comedy is over), and then in a whisper he is said to have muttered, 'I shall hear in Heaven.'

Finally, let me consider the relationship between pulmonary tuberculosis and art and artistic creativity. Pulmonary tuberculosis was very common in the Western world in the eighteenth and nineteenth centuries—as common as it is today in many developing countries. There was no specific treatment, so that progressive tuberculosis meant sure death, at times quickly in a matter of months, invariably within a matter of years. There were many young artists, authors, poets, whose lives and work were cut short by this dreadful disease. Remarkably, there was an impression among many, including doctors, that this disease stimulated creative activity. Perhaps it was a low-grade evening fever observed in many patients, together with a feeling of feverish flush and warmth that led to a dreamy euphoric state. The mind was said to become sharper, associations more vivid, imagination more colourful, so that art, literature, poetry were given an added lustre. There is no scientific proof for this belief, yet there is also no way to disprove it, particularly in those with creative talent. Perhaps it is not the disease but the awareness of slow yet inexorably approaching dissolution which triggers an underlying talent to increased creativity. We will never know.

Among those afflicted with this disease was the poet John Keats, who died of tuberculosis when just 24 years old. Keats had nursed his brother who died of tuberculosis. He had a medical background and when he first coughed up a large quantity of blood he knew he was doomed to die of the disease. In a letter to his fiancée he describes this event—

'I know the colour of that blood, it is arterial blood; I cannot be deceived in that colour, that drop is my death warrant. I must die.'

These were poetic but prophetic words. To be young, to yearn for love and the pleasures of life and yet to know that it will soon be time to die must have been a shattering experience.

In his immortal *Ode to the Nightingale*, the joy, happiness, ecstasy of life are brought out in the Nightingale's wondrous song—

'But being too happy is thy happiness—
That then, light-winged Dryad of the trees,
In some melodious plot
Of beechen green, and shadows numberless,
Singest of summer in full-throated ease'.

Yet the sorrow of existence, his impending dissolution, and the inevitability of death and decay in this world are expressed in exquisite verse.

'Here where men sit and hear each other groan;
Where palsy shakes a few, sad, last grey hairs,
Where youth grows pale and spectre thin and dies;
Where but to think is to be full of sorrow
And leaden-eyed despair,
Where beauty cannot keep her lustrous eyes,
Or new love pine at them beyond tomorrow'.

It was perhaps the bitter thought of approaching death that further sparked his splendid talent and gave wings to his poetic fancy. As tuberculosis consumed him and his end drew near, he developed a serene, extraordinary detachment, a heightened awareness of the beauty and bounty of Nature—'I muse with great affection on every flower I have known since infancy'.

Was it the euphoria caused by tuberculosis, or was it death knocking at the door that set his creative talent on fire? Would this poet-quester ever have chanted his immortal odes to our world if disease and death had not beckoned him at so young an age?

A few of the other greats who suffered from tuberculosis were Anton Chekov, the Bronte sisters, D. H. Lawrence and perhaps Frédéric Chopin.

Chekov contracted tuberculosis at an early age. He was a doctor but refused to accept the diagnosis of his colleagues, though within him he probably knew the truth. His dread of the disease was translated into a number of his works, where again as with Keats, the joy of living on the one hand is countered and quenched by the merciless march of disease and death.

The Bronte sisters were truly cursed with tuberculosis. The two eldest died quickly of the disease. The third Charlotte was left to bring up the two youngest—Emily and Anne, who also died of tuberculosis. Charlotte nursed them right up to the end. The tragedy of her sisters shattered her. Her description of tuberculosis in the chapter 'The Valley of the Shadow of Death' is poetic and of unsurpassed literary beauty. The writings of the Bronte sisters were unquestionably influenced by disease, loneliness, poverty and the bleak, stern background of the barren moors where they lived.

D. H. Lawrence was also a victim of tuberculosis though he tried his best to conceal this both from himself and from others, calling it a chest cold, flu, bronchitis. It is believed that his famous novel, *Lady Chatterley's Lover* was written when he had advanced tuberculosis. Probably the disease also dampened Lawrence's sexual activity, rendering him impotent. Unsatisfied desire could have led to erotic fantasies which were translated into literature, expressing the sexual ecstasies during the physical love between Lady Chatterley and her game-keeper in the novel *Lady Chatterley's Lover.*

Frédéric Chopin's musical genius was nourished by three tragedies. The first and foremost was the tragedy of his exile from his beloved country, Poland, which he left never to return, when just 20 years old. The second was his dreadful disease whose symptoms started at a young age, rendering him increasingly weak, breathless, incapable of exertion. He had recurrent bouts of fever and cough when he spat out blood. It is commonly believed that Chopin's illness denoted tuberculosis. This may have been so, but recent medical theories suggest he may well have suffered from bronchiectasis or cystic fibrosis. In any case the disease ravaged him and resulted in death when he was 39 years old. The third and final tragedy of his life was his tormented love for the author George Sand. All these combined to influence his musical genius. His nocturnes are songs of beauty that whisper dream-like into the silence of a moonlit night; his mazurkas are reminiscent of the Poland he loved and yearned for. His 'Funeral March' is the march of his tragic life—nostalgic memories of happy days in his youth followed by a 'Presto' which has been likened 'to the flutter of the night breeze among tombstones'.

The foregoing pages have shown that in many great artists, ill health and disease have spurred creativity resulting in great art. It is however important to give a balanced overall perspective on the relation between disease and artistic creativity. I shall now do so, and then conclude by recapitulating how creativity arises.

To start with, disease does not necessarily nurture creativity. On the contrary, it may well snuff out artistic talent even before, or soon after it is born. One will never know how many artists have met this unkind fate. Occasionally, disease cuts short brilliant artistic talent. Thus Tennessee Williams's creativity was cut short by alcoholism, while Ernest Hemingway's talent was destroyed by hypertensive disease, alcohol abuse and fits of depression. The genius of Friedrich Nietzsche, the philosopher-poet would have lasted longer had it not been for syphilis affecting the brain, and Maurice Ravel, the French composer would have delighted the world with more of his compositions but for the dementia that afflicted him in his later years. Again, suffering is not necessarily a prerequisite for artistic creativity. An artist does not have to be deaf to compose great music as Beethoven did; or blind to write verse as Milton did; or experience fits of mania to paint as Van Gogh did. A genius at times borders on insanity, but one need not go mad to be considered a genius. Leonardo da Vinci, Michelangelo, Raphael, Pablo Picasso, Henri Matisse, Paul Cezanne, Johanne Sebastian Bach, Wolfgang Amadeus Mozart, Claude Debussy, Igor Stravinski, William Shakespeare, William Wordsworth, T. S. Eliot are just a few of the great artists of the world whose genius was not tempered by serious disease or great suffering. Also, there were and there continue to be many many other artists, perhaps on a slightly lower rung, who have contributed vastly to the artistic treasures of our world and thereby to our joy and happiness.

Yet, we have given ample evidence that in a number of instances, disease or serious ill-health together with the physical and emotional anguish associated with it have sparked artistic creativity and great art. As mentioned earlier, great art always springs from within; it cannot arise from without. In all such artists, suffering, anguish, pain are 'experiences' producing indelible emotions within the subconscious. The French psychoanalyst Jacques Lacan has said that the unconscious is structured like a language—in fact this is the current prevailing concept in modern psychology. I am however more inclined to agree with Freud that the Id, the deepest depth of the unconscious, is unstructured, a whirlpool, a cauldron of emotions, impressions, ideas that result from past 'experiences'. The great artist creates order and gives both form and pattern to these emotions, plucks them out to the conscious level and presents them to the world as great art be it visual art, literature, poetry or music. Great art is transcendental; though personal, it yet transcends the artist. The creative process is not necessarily voluntary, in that it may not be willed by the artist; it can occur unconsciously. It is amazing that though all great creative achievements are products of the human brain, the creative process at least in part may occur at the unconscious level—arising spontaneously through inspiration. The great artist awaits, nay pines for this inspirational force that sets his creativity on fire. Let me once again quote Nietzsche to describe what this great philosopher-poet felt when he was inspired to create *Thus Spoke Zarathustra*.

'... I will describe it;—if one has the slightest residue of superstition left in one, one would hardly be able to set aside the idea that one is merely incarnation, merely mouthpiece, merely medium of overwhelming forces. The concept of revelation in the sense that something suddenly, with unspeakable certainty and subtlety, becomes visible, audible, something that shakes and overturns one to the depths, simply describes the fact.' ... 'Everything is in the highest degree involuntary, but takes place as in a tempest of a feeling of freedom, of absoluteness, of power, of divinity. The involuntary nature of image, of metaphor is the most remarkable thing of all; one no longer has any idea what is image, what metaphor, everything presents itself at the readiest, the truest, the simplest means of expression ... This is my experience of inspiration.'

The meaning of inspiration, of artistic creativity, of the spontaneous involuntary process through which creativity occurs, and the feeling of exhilaration and elation at being 'inspired' to 'create' have no better description in literature.

Great art is life's great treasure; it is an unshakeable counter to an increasingly money-conscious world; it enriches and ennobles life; it enhances the joy of living. It is indeed both a paradox and a mystery of our existence on earth that suffering and anguish can conceivably help create a treasure of such transcendental beauty.

The Story of Anaesthesia

Before me waiting–waiting for the knife,
A little while, and at a leap I storm
The thick, sweet mystery of chloroform,
The drunken dark, the little death in life.

—WILLIAM ERNEST HENLEY

In 2007, the *British Medical Journal* asked its readers to vote on the greatest medical advance since 1840. The discovery of anaesthesia stood a close third on the voter's list, next only to improved sanitation with clean drinking water and antibiotics. Indeed, where would surgery be without the use of anaesthesia? How could the great advances in surgery, the ability of the surgeon today to literally reach out and touch every nook and corner of the human body, to transplant organs, to reshape or correct deformities, ever have been possible without the use of this great discovery?

The scope of surgery right up to the early 1840s was limited. The most limiting factor was pain—nothing had been discovered till then, that could consistently offer relief during a surgical procedure. Surgeons worked with furious speed, as operations had to be completed within a few minutes, else the anguish of unbearable pain could result in shock and death. The other difficult problems that surgeons had to face were haemorrhage, postoperative shock and infection. But the immediate and most pressing problem was the relief of pain.

The frustration in the early 1840s over a situation which seemed to have no solution in sight, led to a trial of unusual methods (not involving drugs) to help in pain relief at surgery. Thus, a new attempt at pain relief was the use of mesmerism to produce oblivion and a state of unconsciousness free of pain. John Elliotson (1791–1868) was the first to use hypnotism in surgical operations. He published his results in 1843. In 1845, John Esdaile, a Scotsman used hypnosis to perform 261 painless surgeries on Hindu prisoners in Bengal. He was rather unsuccessful when he attempted to repeat the performance on his own countrymen in Scotland. These attempts merely indicated the desperateness of the situation which seemed irremediable.

The history of attempts at the pharmacological relief of pain stretches into antiquity. Sleep-inducing drugs included Homer's nepenthe, hemp used in the East, Dioscorides' poison and the mandrake used by the thirteenth century surgeon, Hugh of Lucca. No single drug was consistently effective and right up to the fourth decade of the nineteenth century, a strong dose of opium fortified by an appropriately heavy dose of alcohol was all that could be used. Even so, at the cut of a sharp knife, the agony of surgery became inevitable. Man therefore was reconciled to the idea that what could not be cured had to be endured. This belief was reinforced when it was given a religious connotation in the early years of Christianity. The Church claimed that pain was a visitation from God, a punishment for sins; pain had to be suffered without complaint. Thus it regarded the pain of childbirth as punishment justly inflicted by God. For a woman in childbirth to seek relief from pain was considered a sin punishable by death. There were indeed examples of such women being dragged away from their homes, mercilessly thrown into a pit and buried alive. Religion in this era ran counter to science and the search for pain relief. Yet even if this had not been so, the discovery of anaesthesia would have still remained in the distant future.

What was surgery like in the pre-anaesthetic days? In the first half of the nineteenth century, right up to the 1840s, surgery and surgical techniques were almost the same as in the time of Ambroise Paré in the sixteenth century. The one difference was that the early nineteenth century surgeons were better versed in anatomy and pathology than their colleagues of the Renaissance and Baroque era. Skill, speed and daring remained the prime requisites of surgeons. Brilliance was equated to speed and literally timed by the stop-watch. Sir William Ferguson, one of the top surgeons in London was reported to have said to his students when at work, 'Look out sharp, for if you even wink, you may miss the operation altogether'. The surgeons were like prima donnas at an opera when they strutted into the operating theatre, in fancy street clothes, their surgery being viewed by applauding colleagues, students and outside spectators who thronged the visitor's gallery. There were many great personalities in surgery in the pre-anaesthetic era. In Paris, there was the brilliant Guillaume Dupuytren (1778–1835) who is said to have worn a cloth cap and carpet slippers when operating. In London, besides William Ferguson, there were Astley Cooper, John Hunter, Robert Liston, Benjamin Brodie and James Paget, renowned for their expertise, daring and speed. Perhaps one of the greatest surgeons of the pre-anaesthetic, pre-Listerian era was Ephraim McDowell, a country doctor in the wilds of America who pioneered abdominal surgery by successfully performing an ovariotomy in a woman with a large ovarian tumour.

Then again, what were the hospitals like in the pre-anaesthetic era? The first hospitals that began to emerge in the late eighteenth and early nineteenth century were modelled after the London Hospital built in 1789. The hospital had a huge operating room (like an amphitheatre) on the top floor. There was a bell outside the operating room. It was rung when an operation was contemplated. At the ring of the bell, nurses, physicians, students, orderlies, other aides rushed to the operating room and closed a very heavy door so that the dreadful screams of the patient would not be heard elsewhere. The patient even if sedated had to be held down by several aides and was even gagged if necessary. The operation theatre had a large skylight, so that natural light could stream in and allow the surgeon to see well, considering that electricity was non-existent. The London Hospital was so designed because of the absence of anaesthesia. It became the model for all other hospitals not only in Britain, but also in Europe and America.

With this short preamble of the pre-anaesthetic era, let me now outline the story of the ultimate discovery of anaesthesia, a discovery that revolutionalized surgery enabling it to leap forward to unimagined heights. Every discovery has its precursors. In 1275, Raymundus Lullius, the famous Spanish alchemist discovered that when vitriol (sulphuric acid) was mixed with alcohol and distilled, a sweet white fluid would result. At first Lullius called this fluid sweet vitriol; it was later termed ether. A great and important future awaited this chemical compound; it however took several centuries before its use in surgery was ultimately realized. During the Renaissance, one of its rebels, the Swiss physician Paracelsus used ether in medical patients to relieve severe pain. Paracelsus was no surgeon and the use of ether as an anaesthetic remained untested and undiscovered.

Remarkably enough, the first milestone in the discovery of anaesthesia was not by doctors but by a chemist. In 1772, Priestley discovered nitrous oxide. Priestley was a liberal who championed the cause of the French Revolution. He was also a Methodist minister who then became a dissenting Unitarian minister, espousing rather radical religious beliefs. His radical views on politics and religion aroused the ire of the lords and gentry of London in that age. His house was burnt and he had to flee and seek both political and religious asylum in America.

After Priestley, the pneumatic medicine (medicine by inhalation) that he had founded, caught the fancy of England. A leading exponent of this rather fanciful branch of medicine was Thomas Beddoes of Berkeley, a physician and a chemist. He was a reader in chemistry at Oxford, a neighbour of Jenner whose work on vaccination he initially vehemently opposed and later equally fervently supported. Beddoes, like Priestley was unfortunately also a liberal in a conservative England and was forced to leave his position at Oxford. In 1794 Thomas Beddoes travelled to Bristol and opened the Pneumatic Medicine Institution. Four years later, he appointed Humphry Davy, an exceptional young surgeon-chemist as its superintendent.

Davy who like Jenner faired poorly at school (he left school when he was 13 years old) turned out to be an outstanding man. Without the qualifications to train as a physician, he apprenticed himself to a surgeon-apothecary. He had an enormous interest in chemistry which he learnt on his own. He experimented on himself and on his acquaintances by inhaling nitrous oxide gas. He found that it produced an irresistible desire to laugh and he and his friends would inhale the gas till they would slip into an unconscious state. It was Davy who called nitrous oxide, 'the laughing gas'; he even developed an inhaler through which this gas could be inhaled.

In 1800, Davy produced a remarkable book—the result of his research on the physical, chemical and physiological properties of nitrous oxide. In this book, he recounted how severe pain in his inflamed gum and jaw following the eruption of a wisdom tooth was promptly relieved by the inhalation of nitrous oxide. He wrote, 'As nitrous oxide appears capable of destroying physical pain, it may preferably be used with advantage during surgical operations at which no great effusion of blood takes place.' Not one physician or surgeon in England, on the continent, or in the US took any heed of this observation! Davy too did not pursue this idea and plunged into other meaningful work. This remarkably enough included poetry and chemistry. He was a poet of note and was admired by Coleridge,

Southey and Wordsworth. Coleridge remarked that if Davy had not been the greatest chemist of his age, he would have been the greatest poet. Wordsworth asked Davy to edit the second edition of *Lyrical Ballads* which contained his own poems and the 'Ancient Mariner' by Coleridge. Davy, Coleridge, Southey were all known to inhale nitrous oxide spending some time in laughter and hilarity. Davy's most important work in science was the discovery of the miner's lamp which greatly reduced the risk of explosion in mines. Davy rose to great fame. He could travel safely between London and Paris at the height of the Napoleonic wars, received an award from Napoleon, became a Fellow of the Royal Society at the young age of 25 years and the President of this Society when he was 42 years old. I cannot help feeling he would have earned even more fame and a greater name had he successfully pursued his study on the anaesthetic properties of nitrous oxide.

In 1818, Michael Faraday, the physicist had reported on the pain-relieving properties of inhaled ether. Again, no one took notice.

The focus on the discovery of anaesthesia now shifts to the United States of America. In 1808, William Barton wrote a medical thesis at the University of Pennsylvania confirming Davy's work on nitrous oxide. He too did not develop his idea further. There was a lull of another 30 years before this idea could be put to practical use.

All seemed forgotten when both ether and nitrous oxide were dragged out of oblivion once again not by the medical profession but by show-business. By the 1840s the young people of the US had discovered that they could get 'drunk' by inhaling ether (resulting in what was termed 'ether frolics') or inhaling nitrous oxide (laughing gas parties). The chemists were indeed too happy to supply ether or nitrous oxide and often organized these parties. The party-goers would get jolly, laugh, perform hilarious antics and if they sniffed a bit too much, they would fall into a deep insensible sleep. Quasi-scientific demonstrations in the form of road shows also gained popularity in the United States in the 1830s, and a young lad called

Samuel Colt who wished to promote the revolver which later made him famous, decided to raise money through these shows. Colt came from Hartford, but advertised himself as Doctor Colt of New York, London and Calcutta. He obtained an apparatus that allowed inhalation of nitrous oxide, and in 1832 began staging demonstrations at street corners and on village greens using as his subject any volunteer who was prepared to inhale the gas. The entertainment consisted of strange hilarious antics that the volunteer subjects indulged in after inhaling the nitrous oxide. All went well for young Samuel Colt till one fine day in one of his larger shows he administered the gas to six Indians who promptly fell asleep. Colt realized he was in trouble—for his large audience had not paid to see Indians take a nap. Resourceful as he must have been, he saved the day by persuading a blacksmith in the audience to inhale the gas. The blacksmith fortunately went on rampage, chased Colt all over the stage and then collapsed in a heap on the sleeping Indians, who awoke to find themselves on the floor. The audience felt that they had their money's worth, but Samuel Colt gave up his nitrous oxide demonstrations altogether. Amazingly, in spite of these ether frolics, laughing gas parties, and the quasi-scientific road shows, the significance of insensible sleep produced by nitrous oxide or ether went unnoticed by surgeons.

At last came Crawford Williamson Long (1815-78). He was a young, handsome doctor living and practising at Jefferson in Georgia. Jefferson was a town of just a few hundred people, but Long's practice extended beyond its confines. Long had his University degree from Kentucky and from the University of Pennsylvania, following which he had trained in surgery at New York city before returning to Jefferson, Georgia. He was clever, dedicated and grew increasingly busy in his practice, so much so that he was late at his own marriage because he was busy looking after a very sick patient. He reached the church when almost all the guests had left, thinking that Long had changed his mind and would not turn up! After the ceremony he returned to his patient and did not see his bride for yet another day!

Shortly after the wedding, several of his friends in Jefferson asked him to make nitrous oxide, so that they could have a laughing gas party. Long thought that ether was just as good and made some ether to sniff at the party. The party went off in great jollity. 'Ether frolics' became the rage in Jefferson and in neighbouring towns. At these 'frolics' Long observed that even when hurt and badly bruised while frolicking under the influence of ether, he felt no pain. This was a profound observation and he resolved to put it into practice. He had a patient named James M. Venables who had two tumours on the nape of his neck. Long offered to remove them, promising absence of pain if surgery was done after inhalation of ether. Venables went through the surgery and had one of his tumours removed successfully, experiencing no pain. Ether had been administered just prior to surgery by pouring it on to a towel and letting Venable inhale from it till he became unconscious. The date was 30 March 1842. The doctor's record read thus: James Venables, 1842, administration of ether and removal of tumour—2 dollars. Nine weeks later Long removed the second tumour, again with the same happy, pain-free, successful result. Long continued to give anaesthesia in his surgical practice and by October 1846, when he was just 26 years old, he had administered surgical anaesthesia successfully to eight patients. He was also the first to use anaesthesia in an obstetric procedure in 1845.

Unfortunately, Crawford Long made no announcement of his discovery, nor did he write to a medical journal or a recognized colleague of his work. He thus failed to offer his work to the medical fraternity. Rightly or wrongly, this detracted from his claim to fame, and from what would have been an otherwise indisputable right to be considered as the man who discovered surgical anaesthesia. Indeed, Long made known his results only in 1849, after he had used ether several times in surgery and after its effectiveness had already been proved by Morton and others. Perhaps he would have continued as before in splendid isolation, but was prompted to write his results in 1849 only when he was aware of the dispute in the claims to fame for the discovery of anaesthesia made by others in the field.

Let me now go on to another personality vying for the honour of being considered the discoverer of anaesthesia. He was Horace Wells (1815-48), a dentist who graduated from the Harvard Dental School in 1834 and who taught dentistry for several years at Harvard. He was gifted but was reported to be an unstable individual. He had temporarily given up his dental practice at one stage, to buy art in France and sell it at a profit. He was noted to be religious and often depressed. In December, Wells attended one of these laughing parties given by Dr G. Colton. He sat next to an individual who had inhaled laughing gas; this man had a severely bruised leg but felt no pain. Wells requested Dr Colton to supply him with nitrous oxide, as he felt that a tooth could be extracted painlessly under the effect of the gas. Colton agreed, accompanied Wells to his office, administered the nitrous oxide gas to Wells, while a colleague pulled out one of Wells's teeth. Wells is said to have exclaimed 'It is the greatest discovery ever made! I did not feel so much as a prick of a pin'. Wells felt certain he was on his way to a big fortune!

Wells was also eager for fame; he was a man in a tearing hurry—and the thought of fame and fortune haunted him. He had an assistant named William Thomas Green Morton who had enrolled as a student in medicine at Harvard. Morton perhaps tried to dissuade him from being overhasty. Wells did not listen and had Morton arrange a demonstration of the discovery of nitrous oxide as an anaesthetic agent at the Massachusetts General Hospital. One of the students volunteered to have a bad tooth extracted and Wells made him inhale the gas. But there was a fiasco. Almost certainly the apparatus he used did not allow the necessary volume of gas to be inhaled so as to produce an anaesthetic effect. As Wells pulled the tooth out, the patient let out a yell of pain. There was pandemonium in the lecture hall and poor Wells dropped his instruments and fled. Wells was devastated and sank into deep depression. He however continued his dental practice and used laughing gas (nitrous oxide) successfully as an anaesthetic on 40 patients during his dental procedures. He had witnesses to this effect for each dental procedure. Unfortunately, no one at the Massachusetts General Hospital believed him.

We now turn to the last two important dramatis personae to complete the story of anaesthesia. They were William Thomas Green Morton and Charles Jackson. Morton besides assisting Wells at dentistry was as mentioned earlier a medical student at Harvard. Charles Jackson, a brilliant physician at Harvard, was Morton's preceptor. There now developed an unfortunate association between the two, an association which bred antagonism and which ultimately led to confusion, confrontation and conflict that baffled even the US House of Congress.

Jackson supplied Morton with ether and suggested that he use it to relieve pain at surgery. Morton felt that if ether fumes were inhaled steadily, ether might be the analgesic for which he was searching. He promptly decided to experiment and his experiments started at home. He took his wife Elizabeth and her spaniel dog Wig for a holiday. Surreptitiously, he made the unwilling dog inhale ether and Wig went into a senseless slumber from which he could be aroused with difficulty. Next in line were the family goldfish who went into a splendid slumber after inhaling ether. His wife Elizabeth was distraught at this scene but was pacified when Morton threw them back into the water, apparently unhurt. Finally, Elizabeth found Morton himself stretched out on the floor—he had inhaled enough ether to knock himself unconscious; even the hysterics of his wife failed to hasten his awakening. Morton and family now returned to Boston and Morton continued his experiments using ether on patients who needed dental extraction; to start with these were not uniformly successful. He consulted Jackson once again, though by now they were not on friendly terms. Jackson advised that the ether Morton used was commercially prepared and impure; pure ether was required, and they should make pure ether on their own. This they did, mixed the pure ether with aromatic oils and called the concoction *Letheon*. They patented this in the hope that if successful, they could earn a fortune!

Morton was now prepared to use *Letheon* on the next patient who required dental extraction. Eben Frost, a musician, walked into Morton's clinic for a painful tooth needing extraction. Morton and his assistant (a dentist named Hayden) got to work. Morton soaked a handkerchief with *Letheon*, held it to Frost's nose to render him unconscious. Hayden focused a lamp very near to Morton to help him with his procedure, and providentially did not blow up the clinic (neither knew that ether was highly inflammable). The dental extraction was successful and painless. Frost became Morton's ardent disciple, his prize exhibit. Morton now felt ready to use ether for surgical operations. He therefore first decided to design an inhaler. He then decided to meet Dr John Collin Warren, the most famous and senior surgeon of the Massachusetts General Hospital, who agreed to allow Morton to use his anaesthetic agent on a patient fixed for surgery. The patient for surgery was Gilbert Abbott, who had a tumour in the neck behind the jaw. The day and time of surgery were notified to Morton, as also to faculty members, residents and students of the hospital.

The morning of the appointed day arrived—Friday 16 October, 1846. The patient was wheeled in—a pale, consumptive-looking young man with a large tumour behind the jaw being taken to the operation table. Then entered Dr Warrren, who explained briefly to the audience as to what was about to take place. The tiers in the theatre were packed with faculty members, doctors and students. There was a silence after his talk. It was a quarter hour past the time fixed for surgery. There now arose a titter among the spectators which became louder with time. Sarcastic comments on the absence of Morton were heard. Dr Warren then spoke: 'Since Dr Morton has not appeared, I presume he is otherwise engaged'. He held up his knife and bent over the patient, ready to begin. Just then the door burst open and Morton appeared, totally out of breath. He was accompanied by his prize exhibit Eben Frost. Morton explained that his delay was due to his inhalation apparatus not being ready on time, but that he was now well equipped and ready to begin. Warren after hearing him, replied a trifle sarcastically, 'Well Sir, your patient is ready'. Morton went to the head of the table and reassured the patient, pointing to Eben Frost who testified to the successful use of ether vapour on himself. Amidst tense silence, the patient followed Morton's instruction. The glass tube of the instrument was inserted into the mouth and he inhaled deeply and evenly. He began to breathe faster, was flushed in the face but then lay quietly sleeping on the operation table. Morton now looked at Dr Warren and said, 'Doctor, your patient is ready'. In the silence of that eventful morning, Dr Warren picked up his scalpel and went to work. The tumour was removed and the wound sutured. Towards the end, Abbott who all that while had laid still, stirred, uttering incoherent sounds, but on recovering consciousness admitted that he felt no pain. Warren was deeply moved, and turning to the spectators muttered, 'Gentlemen, this is no humbug'.

At the next operation, Morton again anaesthetized a patient who had a large tumour in his left arm. The operation was successful; the patient lay unconscious all through surgery and experienced no pain. Warren now promptly ordered the inhalation apparatus and the *Letheon* (which really was ether with aromatic oils) for hospital use. He was told that this was not possible as both Morton and Jackson had acquired patent rights for both. The Massachusetts Medical Society on hearing this was deeply incensed. They declared it was unethical to allow a discovery or an invention that could benefit mankind to be used for private profit and that if an amicable arrangement was not arrived at, the society would ban its use. They were doubly incensed when they learnt that *Letheon* was in essence pure ether and that it had been so named with profit as the main motive. Warren conveyed these views of the Massachusetts Medical Society to Morton, who to his credit wrote the following letter to Warren: 'Dear Sir, as it may sometime be desirable that surgical operations should be performed at Massachusetts General Hospital under the influence of the preparation employed by me for producing temporary insensibility to pain, you will allow me, through you, to offer to the hospital the free use of it for all hospital operations.'

In November 1846, Dr J. H. Bigelow, a colleague in the surgical unit, published reports of Morton's two successful cases in the Boston Medical and Surgical Journal. Within a month of this publication ether was being used in London. The surgeon was Robert Liston, the operation being an amputation. When the patient regained consciouness and realized that he had felt no pain during surgery, he dropped back on the operation table weeping with relief. Liston turned to the students and doctors in the theatre and said, 'This Yankee dodge, gentlemen, beats Mesmer hollow'. Ether thus became popular all over Europe and was in wide use by the end of 1846. Remarkably enough, probably the first lady anaesthetist in the world according to a recent publication of the Indian Journal of Anaesthesia was Dr Ms Roopa Furdoonji, a Parsi lady who worked in Hyderabad, India, in 1889.

The new discovery needed a name. It was Oliver Wendell Holmes who finally gave the acceptable name of '*anaesthesia*'. The term in fact was the ancient Greek word used by Plato and Dioscorides and meant *insensitivity*. Dioscorides' potion, used in antiquity to relieve pain was made thus: boil roots of mandrake in wine until the liquid is reduced to one-third; then administer the decoction in a cup to a patient before operation or cauterization, so that the patient is in a state of *insensitivity*. Mandrake contained alkaloid which like hemp and poppy was used in antiquity for relief of pain. These drugs were banned in the Dark and Middle Ages because they proved dangerous and could cause death.

The sequel to the story of anaesthesia now turned sordid. Who then discovered anaesthesia? Morton, Jackson, Wells, Long were all in contention. A continuing controversy did not help matters. The House of Congress debated this for 16 years despite the onset of the Civil War, but came to no conclusion. Morton gave up his practice to study and publicize the use of ether anaesthesia in surgery, impoverishing himself in the bargain. His torment that the recognition due to him continued to be debated added to his distress. Morton sank from poverty to penury but managed to rescue his house at Wellesley from creditors and supported himself by farming. He died in July 1868 when only 48 years old.

Of the four claimants, undoubtedly Charles Jackson was the cleverest, yet the most devious and untrustworthy. He maintained that he taught Morton all that was to be known about ether and had instructed him on its use. He claimed that once when a bad throat infection had caused him severe pain, he had inhaled ether on his own and had fallen into a painless deep slumber. He dated this incident even before Crawford Long operated on Venables under ether. But was he to be believed? His colleagues remembered him as deceitful, manipulative, with sociopathic tendencies. At many times in his career he had falsely claimed a number of discoveries which in fact had been made by others. Remarkably, Harvard had neither bothered nor disciplined him over these indiscretions. While the controversy on the discovery of anaesthesia was still raging, Jackson became demented and remained so for the rest of his life.

As for Horace Wells, though his demonstration at the Massachusetts General Hospital was a fiasco, he did indeed use nitrous oxide successfully subsequently in many dental operations, though not in general surgical procedures. Wells soon after sank into a state of deep depression, perhaps triggered by the lack of recognition of his claim. He committed suicide by opening a vein and inhaling ether.

Crawford Long undoubtedly was the first to use ether as an anaesthetic—only he did not report it. He was unquestionably the greatest gentleman of the four. He continued to practise surgery and anaesthesia, unruffled by the debate raging around him; as if it were of no consequence. He died suddenly from a massive cerebral haemorrhage while delivering a baby of a local congressman's wife. His dying words were: 'Care for the mother and child first.'

Besides the House of Congress which came to no conclusion even after 16 years of discussion, various medical societies also debated the question as to who discovered anaesthesia—and came to different opinions. The American Dental Association and the American Medical Association gave the honour to Horace Wells. In 1913, the electors of the New York University Hall of Fame considered this issue at great length and concluded that William Thomas Green Morton was the discoverer of anaesthesia. In this debate at the New York University, the most famous participant was Sir William Osler who chose Morton in favour of Long and convinced the electors of the University to do likewise. His argument was that 'in science credit should go to the one who reports his work and convinces the world, not to the one who first has an idea or who proves that this idea works.'

However, the American College of Surgeons at a meeting in Atlanta in 1923 gave the distinction to Crawford Long and created the Crawford Long Association, which in 1926 erected a statue of Long at Statutory Hall in Washington DC. Later, a hospital in Atlanta was named the Long Memorial Hospital. Most surgeons now accept Long as the discoverer of anaesthesia.

I shall now conclude the story of anaesthesia with a brief description of the use of chloroform, an anaesthetic agent, which came into use soon after ether. Sir James W. Simpson, the Scottish obstetrician had used ether with great success but was dissatisfied because of its strong smell and the bronchial irritation it often caused. He therefore experimented with chloroform, a new anaesthetic described by the American Samuel Guthrie in 1832. He used chloroform to ease the pain of pregnant mothers during labour. This brought the wrath of the Scottish clergy upon him. Labour pains according to the clergy were ordained by God. Did not the book of Genesis state, 'with pangs shall you give birth to children'? Simpson cleverly responded that the book also stated that God made Adam fall asleep before taking a rib from him to create Eve. God therefore anaesthetized Adam. The medical profession in Philadelphia sided with the clergy, stating that the pain of childbirth was a natural and necessary manifestation and should not be relieved. Simpson, not to be outdone, replied that when they next wished to travel to New York, they should walk, as it was a natural thing to do and not take the train! These polemics did not however help the use of anaesthesia in childbirth. It was only when Queen Victoria gave her royal assent to chloroform anaesthesia for the delivery of Prince Leopold, her seventh child, that anaesthesia using chloroform became fashionable and acceptable. Her obstetrician was John Snow and his work on chloroform and other anaesthetics gave anaesthesia an increasingly scientific basis.

Technical developments in the discovery of newer anaesthetic agents and in their administration kept apace. The story of anaesthesia continues spilling over into the period of contemporary and modern medicine. The anaesthetist has evolved from a scared individual pouring an unknown quantity of ether on to a handkerchief and later a face-mask placed on the patient's nose and mouth, to a highly-trained individual practising a quickly-evolving speciality. He can today maintain the patient at any level of consciousness desired by the surgeon; he can collapse a lung when necessary and re-inflate it at the appropriate time. He controls a formidable array of dials and has a number of instruments at his command to monitor the effect of one or more anaesthetics he administers. He intervenes with appropriate drugs when vital signs change, and he works in tandem with the surgeon for the greater glory of surgery.

But who started it all? Was it Crawford Long, the country surgeon, a gentleman working in isolation in Jefferson, a very small town in Georgia in the US, or was it the dentist Horace Wells at Harvard, was it the deceitful but very clever Charles Jackson, or was it the lucky William Thomas Green Morton, who successfully demonstrated the use of ether as an anaesthetic, before an august assembly of doctors at the premier university of the United States? The *British Medical Journal* should now seek a vote from its readers on this issue.

Religion and Medicine

And almost every one when age,
Disease or sorrows strike him,
Inclines to think there is a God,
Or something very like him.

—Arthur Hugh Clough

It was around 6000 years ago that man emerged from the shadows of the Stone Age into the first light of civilization and into recorded history. The great ancient civilizations of the past were established along the banks of mighty rivers—Mesopotamia on the hot dusty plains between the rivers Euphrates and Tigris, Egypt along the verdant and marshy banks of the river Nile, India along the banks of the mighty Indus and China along the banks of the Yellow river. It is possible that these river valleys provided the right challenge to elicit the maximal creative response from man. The challenge did not overwhelm him into defeat, nor was it so dull as to lull him into a torpor of inactivity. It provided the right impetus so that a succession of challenges called forth a succession of responses culminating into the first great civilizations of history.

In the early centuries of these civilizations of antiquity, medicine was a blend of magic and religion—magic, inseparably mixed with religious beliefs. It is not difficult to comprehend why this should be so. The book of civilization must have opened with early man intrigued, befuddled, and often frightened at what he saw and experienced. The sun, the moon, the stars and the canopy of the sky above him, the floods of mighty rivers, the changing seasons, natural disasters in the form of drought, storms, earthquakes, defied the explanations of ancient man. The mystery of life, of disease, of birth and the annihilation into nothingness caused by death, for which even today man has no answer, must have caused awe, anguish and fear. These were challenges early man could neither defeat nor defy, yet he had to offer a response. Much of what he saw, felt and experienced, seemed without obvious cause, seemed unnatural; he therefore responded by believing in supernatural causes to the inexplicable aspects of life and living. Thereby came the entry of numerous gods and of religion into the world of man.

In the early centuries of all these ancient civilizations it was believed that disease was caused by evil spirits, both supernatural and earthly that entered through the body orifices wreaking havoc within the victim. The purpose of medicine was to rid the body of these demons. The approach was in the form of supplications, incantations, the casting of magic spells and the practice of magical rituals. To start with, medicine in this form was practised by the shamans of ancient Egypt, Sumer, and other civilizations of antiquity. Then came on to the scene the priest who combined with his priestly role the duty of a physician. The chief priest physicians of the King of Sumer or the Pharaohs of Egypt wielded immense power and influence.

In ancient Egypt, cures for diseases were revealed by the gods, and these cures were categorized by Thoth, the Ibis-headed god of wisdom in secret books. These secret books were guarded in the medical schools associated with the temples of Sais at Heliopolis. They formed the medical texts for the priest physicians of Egypt.

It was Thoth who knew the secrets of all the gods and could cause and cure all disease. Other popular gods to whom supplications were addressed or incantations recited were the falcon-headed sun-god Ré and the goddess Isis with her son Horus, the god of health. The gods could cure but could also exert magic capable of killing an individual. In many primitive communities in different parts of the world, casting a curse through sympathetic magic is practised even today. Catherine de Medici of Austria who became the Queen of France in AD 1559 was said to be a devotee of this form of magic. Hair, clothing, or nail parings from the intended victim were mixed with wax into a figure that resembled the victim. When the figurine was cursed the victim succumbed to an illness and died.

In addition to religio-medical practices there now evolved over time the practice of empirical medicine—medicine based on observation and experience. Even today, a great deal of modern medicine is empirical, a practice that originated well over 5000 years ago. While in the earlier dynasties the physician was a priest, in the later period he attained an independent professional status. There were now three forms of practice—the shaman who practised sorcery and magic to cure disease, the priest physician with his religio-magical practice who also claimed to specialize in disease, and the professional physician who did not necessarily eschew religio-medical beliefs but who introduced the practice of empirical medicine. As centuries rolled by in the civilization of Egypt, the professional physician grew to be a man of wide learning and culture, steeped in the lore of centuries and possessed of a sound knowledge of empiric medicine.

Information on the content of Egyptian medicine is obtained from Greek and Roman manuscripts and most important of all from a study of medical papyri. The most important of these papyri are the Edwin Smith papyrus (1600 BC) found near Luxor and the George Ebers papyrus (1580 BC) from Thebes. The Edwin Smith papyrus though written around 1600 BC, describes medical practice of even earlier times. The George Ebers papyrus is a collection of medical texts which probably originated in the old empire (3300–2600 BC), during the time of the first eight dynasties whose Pharaohs expressed their might and glory by building the Pyramids of Cheops, Chefren and Mycerinus. The Ebers papyrus is perhaps the oldest surviving treatise on medicine. Over 20 metres long, it deals with magic cum religious healing as also with empiric medicine.

From the mists of antiquity, about 2700 BC, there emerged for the first time in recorded history the detailed description of the vivid personality of a great physician. His name was Imhotep (he who cometh in peace). He was indeed a priest physician, the high priest at Heliopolis, as also the grand vizier and architect to the Pharaoh Zoser. He was a multifaceted personality, and must have been truly gifted, for he was renowned also as a sage, astronomer, scribe, but above all as a great physician—wise, learned and kind. When he died, Egypt wept—people lined the banks of the Nile in grief as his body was being taken down the river in a ceremonial barge. The link between religion and medicine, was even more strongly forged, when within a few generations he was deified, so that by the sixth century BC he had displaced Thoth as the God of healing in Egypt and had even been given a divine father, the God Ptah. The Greeks in time to come identified him with Askelepius, more commonly known today by his Latin name Aesculapius, their God of medicine. It is possible that Imhotep after his death was associated with healing temple shrines in ancient Egypt, just as Askelepius the Greek god came to be associated with temple shrines in Greece. The cult of Askelepius the Greek god, in time fused with the Egyptian Imhotep to become the cult of Askelepius-Imhotep.

The link between medicine and religion was equally strong in ancient Sumer, India and China as it was in Egypt. Each of these civilizations of antiquity gave their own names to their own set of numerous gods, allocating each god different powers and functions. These were however just minor variations to a common central theme of magic cum religious healing, embellished later, with empiricism.

There was however one civilization in the Middle East which needs special mention—the civilization of ancient Persia. Before the seventh century BC, the Persians believed in a pantheon of numerous gods as did all members of the Indo-European race. Their priests were the Magi who brought animal sacrifices to the gods, and like all religions of contemporary and early civilizations laid stress on magic, rituals, and supernatural forces to aid healing. Then there came a prophet, a reformer, an enlightened soul, Zoroaster or Zarathustra. According to Greek historians he preached in Persia in the seventh and sixth century BC. Modern Oriental and Persian scholars however believe that he lived as far back as 1200 BC, attacking and denouncing the pantheon of old traditional gods. He preached that there was just one God, Ahura Mazda, omnipotent, omniscient, the creator, the source of light, truth, purity and righteousness.

The tenets of Zoroastrianism remain amazingly simple and practical. They are embodied in the three words—humata, hukata, havarashta—which mean good thoughts, good words and good deeds. Righteousness is the essence of the religion, but it should be righteousness for the sake of righteousness. Unquestionably, the greatest gift of Persia to mankind was that it gave birth to the first monotheistic religion in the world—Zoroastrianism. The concept of one God, of good and evil and of man's obligation to choose between the two, between God and the Devil, between Heaven and Hell found its way into all subsequent monotheistic religions— Judaism, Christianity and Islam. Though Zoroastrianism abolished the pantheon of gods of early and contemporary civilization, substituting this pantheon with one God, the practice of medicine remained closely linked to religion. Thus Zoroastrian scriptures (the Avesta) are the main source of our knowledge on the practice of medicine in ancient Persia. Empirical medicine (as in all earlier civilizations) was slowly gaining root, yet incantations and prayers to the one God remained an important form of medical practice. Of all practising physicians, the priest-physician was considered the wisest and the most capable. The power of prayers to aid healing of the sick and the ailing remained paramount. Let me quote from the Avestan scriptures:

'Of all the healers O Spitama Zarathustra, namely those, who heal with the knife, with herbs and with sacred incantations, the last one is the most potent as he heals from the source of disease' (Ardibest Yasht).

Civilization in the West and the Changing Features of Medicine

Egypt declined after 27 centuries of unbroken splendour and the heart of civilization moved from the heat and dust of the lands of the Middle East to the craggy shores of the Greek peninsula, to the glittering sunlit islands afloat on the Aegean sea and to the coast of Asia Minor which had witnessed the ebb and flow of earlier civilizations. Nature posed a different kind of challenge which evoked a different and even more brilliant response than the civilizations which preceded it. Classical Greece is rightly perceived as the mother of Western civilization and the cradle of the human spirit. No longer was man a pitiable plaything or pawn at the mercy of tyrants. He was a being of great worth, capable of great thought and action. The Greeks had their own pantheon of gods. Man was made in the image of their gods—only he was mortal.

Greece posed eternal questions to the world. What is nature and who is Man? Where does he come from and where does he go? From this debate and the curiosity of the human spirit to understand man and nature was born philosophy and out of philosophy was born medicine.

Pythagoras, the philosopher scientist founded his school of philosophy on the southern coast of Italy. Philosophy, science and medicine became closely related fields; they grew out of the curiosity to know more about man and his environment. Thus just as the roots of medicine in the civilizations of antiquity were magic and religion, the roots of medicine in the evolving Western civilization in Greece were philosophy and science. Even so, in the first five hundred years before Christ, there flourished two different schools of medicine in Greece—the school believing in the cult of Aesculapius (a school of religion and faith) and the rational school of medicine as taught by the great Hippocrates and his followers. There then began a tussle between religion and rationality, between faith and science—a conflict which persists even in our present age. Let me briefly describe these two opposing schools of medicine.

The Religious School—The Cult of Aesculapius

The Cult of Aesculapius or Askelepius perhaps originated from the worship of the presiding deities of the underworld, Pluto, Prosperine or Cereberus who had the power to cure or avert disease. Legendary powers of healing were attributed to Aesculapius, but it is impossible to determine if Aesculapius really lived and practised as a doctor as did Imhotep of Egypt or whether he was a legendary figure. He was mythically born of the Greek god Apollo and the nymph Corona. Her flirtation with a mortal aroused the ire of Apollo who killed the nymph with his arrow. But in death the god delivered her of an infant son, Aesculapius. Aesculapius was taught the art of healing by the kind wine centaur Chiron. He grew up to be a great and kind doctor who had the supernatural power to raise the dead. Pluto, the prime deity of the underworld felt that his domain would in time be underpopulated and complained to the gods. Thereupon, Jupiter struck Aesculapius dead with a thunderbolt and carried him up to the abode of the gods at Mount Olympus. Legend has it that Aesculapius then returned to earth as a hero among mortals.

Aesculapius was worshipped in beautifully designed temples all over Greece. The temples were set in lively pastoral surroundings, with gardens, bathing pools, gymnasiums and spas. Around this figure rose a cult of medicine which attracted the ill and afflicted in thousands from all corners of Greece. A number of these temples (starting from before 770 BC) began to dot the Greek landscape.

Numerous miracles and cures were said to have been performed in these Aesculapian temples—all were attributed to Aesculapius, the god of healing. Cures and miracles were recorded on tablets hung on the walls of temples. Miraculous cures of the dumb speaking after a night's sojourn in the Aesculapian temple, of the paralyzed walking out at daybreak, of women condemned to infertility conceiving, are all recorded for posterity on votive tablets which were presented by grateful devotees. There must perhaps have been some chicanery, hypocrisy or greed involved in the working of these temples, but healing through faith is not to be scorned or laughed at. It persists to this day at the many religious shrines of which Lourdes in France and Tirupati, Vaishnodevi and several other temples and shrines in India are outstanding examples. There also exist even today a large number of shrines in India, the Far East, Africa, Russia and other parts of Europe, where devotees gather to be blessed and healed.

The Hippocratic School—The School of Rational Medicine

In the fifth century BC, Greek medicine was epitomized by Hippocrates, the Father of Medicine. Hippocrates was born on the island of Cos around 470 BC. By this time of course, the cult of Aesculapius which was prevalent from around 700 BC onwards had taken root. Thus the cult of Aesculapius and the Hippocratic School of Rational Medicine were practised concurrently from the fifth century BC onwards, for several hundred years.

Hippocrates taught medicine to his students and followers under a big plane tree on the island of Cos. His conception of disease was arresting. Of utmost importance, he broke the link between medicine and religion. He thus expelled the gods and their role in the causation and cure of disease. Disease, Hippocrates claimed, was due to natural causes; supernatural effects had no role to play in the practice of medicine. Medicine should be rational so that the causes, effects and the cure of disease were explicable on a natural and rational basis. Let me give just one example of Hippocratic teaching. Epilepsy was till then supposed to be a 'sacred' and 'divine' disease. This is what Hippocrates had to say on epilepsy. 'I am about to discuss the disease called sacred (epilepsy). It is not in my opinion any more divine or more sacred than other disease, but has a natural cause, and its supposed divine origin is due to man's inexperience, and their wonder at its peculiar character.'

The writings of Hippocrates have been collected together in the *Corpus Hippocraticum*. They number about 72 texts and over 50 treatises, documenting the medical knowledge of the times. These collections were assembled in the third century BC, in the great library of Alexandria, at the behest of Ptolemy, one of Alexandria's generals who ruled Egypt after the death of Alexander. The *Corpus Hippocraticum* included works on medicine, surgery, gynaecology, obstetrics, public health and hygiene, dietetics, and the role of environmental disease.

One of the greatest attributes of Hippocrates and his teachings was on the practice of bedside medicine, and on the art of observation of the natural history of disease. The art of diagnosis was related to a holistic understanding of the patient's character, diet, habits and lifestyle, to a meticulous bedside history-taking and to an astute power of observation, through the use of eyes, ears and the hands. Treatment was empirical, but Hippocrates emphasized on the healing powers of nature. 'Nature heals—assist it'. Perhaps even greater than the medical texts of the *Corpus Hippocraticum* was the code of ethics laid down by Hippocrates. It was said to be recited under a great plane tree on the island of Cos by all young men who were formally initiated into the art and science of medicine. There are some who believe that the oath was not a part of his teachings, but was a Pythagorean concept that was added to the *Corpus Hippocraticum* in later years.

This description of the Hippocratic school has been given to illustrate the paradigm shift in the practice of medicine. It is the consistency of the rational approach and the total exclusion of all other approaches, as also the emphasis on humanism and humanity within the core of his teachings that make Hippocratic medicine a great landmark in the history of man and medicine.

The rivalry between the cult of Aesculapius and Hippocratic medicine continued well into the fourth century AD, coming to an end only when the Christian emperor Constantine demolished the last temple of Aesculapius in Aegae, Wesia during his reign (331–337). Thus it was the Hippocratic school of rational medicine that ultimately triumphed. This is because the spirit of free thought which allowed intelligent criticism in all spheres of activity, be it religion or art or politics, was one of the basic tenets of Greek civilization. Independent minds saw through at least some of the chicanery that passed for Aesculapian healing in many of these temples. The essence of Greek civilization was the free spirit of inquiry. A priestly religion or a religio-medical cult involved supernatural forces and the Greek mind could not readily accept forces which could neither be observed nor measured. This is the reason why the objective and philosophical schools of lay medicine triumphed over the Aesculapian cult.

Christianity and Medicine

Though Rome conquered Greece, it was Greece which in essence captured Rome, for it was the civilization of Greece which either permeated or influenced life and living in the Roman empire. The Roman empire at its zenith spread far and wide—far west to include Britain, Spain and Gaul, and east to include Egypt, Asia minor, Persia, right up to the border of India. Great though Rome's achievements were in law, administration, public works, technology and feat of arms, Rome lacked the graciousness, the spirit of freedom, loftiness of thought and action, displayed by Greece. Yet Rome gave the Western world the PAX ROMANA for several hundred years, a feat unrivalled till the present day. But Rome like all great civilizations ultimately declined and fell. Aleric the Goth, delivered the coup de grace when he pillaged and sacked Rome in AD 410.The official death-knell of the Western Roman empire was tolled in AD 476 when Emperor Romulus Augustus was deposed by Odacear, King of the barbaric Herulians. Those familiar with Gibbon's *Decline and Fall of the Roman Empire* would attribute its fall to the rise of Christianity. It is inferred that Christianity divided loyalties. Rome was great when its undivided loyalty was for the state and what it stood for. Rome declined and fell when its loyalties were divided between religion and state, with a greater preference for religion than the state. Thus the coming of Christ perhaps sounded the death-knell of Rome.

But this is not entirely true. Rome fell because it had become rotten to the core. She committed a thousand crimes, worshipped the cult of force and violence, practised barbaric cruelty, trampled upon the poor, taxed the impoverished to support the luxury of the rich and failed to protect its citizens from famine, disease and death. There was a canker eating into its soul and tearing apart its body politic. The barbarian onslaught from without and Christianity from within were not the root causes of Rome's fall; they merely hastened its decline and death.

The fall of Rome was however a catastrophe, introducing the Dark Ages which stretched almost up to the Renaissance. Law and order collapsed; anarchy prevailed. Pestilence, famine and war stalked the Western world. Plague and smallpox decimated communities, villages and cities within a few days or weeks. How could man believe in or trust any form of medicine when he was witness to rampant death and disease?

The lamp of learning and that of all human endeavour was extinguished. In this dark and savage era there was however a glimmer of hope. This glimmer was the birth of Christianity preceded by the coming of Christ. Christ, Christianity and the churches that grew out of Christianity offered 'Faith' as the supreme healing power. Religion and faith became once more the core of medicine.

It is of interest to briefly consider the outlook of Christianity on disease and on healing. Christianity considered man to have a body which was temporary and a soul which was eternal. The priest ministered to the eternal soul and was superior to the physician who ministered to the physical body. The 'eternal' obviously took precedence over the 'temporary' though the borders between the two were at times indistinct. Even so, the physician and the priest over a period of centuries learnt to respect each other and lived in happy symbiosis.

The concept of disease held by Christianity was partly influenced by earlier religions like the Egyptian religion and the Old Testament of the Jews and was partly original in its flavour. Disease was thus considered as a punishment for sins as in the Old Testament, or as a visitation of the wrath of God. Egyptian and Mesopotamian beliefs were similar, except these civilizations believed in many gods while both Jewish and Christian religions were monotheistic. An unusual concept of disease in Christianity was that disease could be a God-given trial to those He loved and who after death would reap the bounty of perpetual bliss in paradise. Christianity's attitude to medicine was embodied in the tenet that healing was its mission. It regarded medicine and the care of the poor, the sick and afflicted as a work of charity. This religious belief reaped a tremendous advantage and immeasurable goodwill when it proclaimed that helping the sick was a boundless duty for both the individual and the community. It was not an empty proclamation; it was put into effect with zeal and devotion. Medicine after the fall of Rome and in the Dark Ages was thus usurped by the church and given a strongly religious flavour. Healing was through faith, through inviting the help of God, the Father. The use of holy oil, prayer, 'laying of hands' helped to heal better than the medicaments of the Egyptian or Greco-Roman Age.

The healing power of faith was demonstrated in the gospel. Jesus Christ performed miracles by healing, involving the help of God, the

Father—the blind could see, the lame could walk, the leper became free of his dreadful scourge. There are more than 30 miraculous cures recorded in the Bible; healing was considered by the apostles of Christ as a 'gift of the spirit'. It is understandable that the numerous sick, diseased individuals in the Dark Ages turned to Christianity both for physical cure and for eternal salvation. Men, women, children and even infants in arms would wait patiently for baptism, anointment with holy oil or the use of some holy relic to bring relief to their suffering bodies. Christian shrines, where the act of healing through faith and prayer became popular, were established—often on the ruins of old pagan temples. Two of the first Christian doctors who practised healing by faith were Cosmos and Damian. They suffered martyrdom and were later beatified.

Christianity may well be considered as an important cause of the decline of medicine and of a temporary end to the spirit of scientific inquiry. But then, a religion is more concerned with the promotion of its religious doctrines than with speculation and research either in medicine or on the natural sciences. Perhaps a more appropriate view is that medicine, science and the liberal arts all declined through default in an age riven by disorder and strife. Even so, Christianity did a great deal to relieve suffering in difficult times. Hospices called Xenodochia were built at different sites, affording food and shelter to the poor and the pilgrims; in later years these were converted into hospitals. Christian charity was first institutionalized in the Eastern Empire as a sequel to Constantine's recognition of Christianity as the official religion of the state. The bishop of Antioch first set up hospitals in his see. The first great Christian hospital was built in the Eastern Empire by St. Basil at Caesarea in the year AD 370. The hospital was like a township with as many wards as there were diseases. Charity, love, compassion were also extended to lepers who from time immemorial had been kept in isolation. St. Basil's hospital also included a leper colony, where the inmates were cared for with true dedication. It needs be mentioned that the first hospital in the

Western world was built by the Roman Lady Fabiola in AD 394. She suffered two unhappy marriages, became the follower of St. Jerome and did penance in the Chalcis desert from where she returned in AD 381. She devoted herself to the sick and poor, spending her wealth on charity.

Thus when Hippocratic and Galenic medicine well-nigh perished, Christianity substituted the practice of medicine with the power of faith. It helped preserve and perpetuate the Hippocratic tenet of care and devotion to the sick and afflicted. It provided first for retreats and then for hospitals all over Christendom.

There was one other very important way in which the Christian faith and religion related not only to medicine but to the fruits of all other human endeavours. Having withstood and triumphed over the turbulence of this unsettled age, the realization dawned on Christianity and the Christian church that it owed a duty to itself and to the world to preserve the achievements of the Greco-Roman past, and to save them from being annihilated forever. Christianity built numerous monasteries all over Europe and even the Middle East. It was within the confines of churches and monasteries that precious manuscripts and documents on medicine and other subjects were carefully hidden and thereby preserved from the fury of marauders and rampaging mobs.

To provide a more balanced view, I will now briefly highlight some of the exaggerated claims as also undesirable effects that Christianity had in this historical era. The claim often made, that Christianity furthered learning and established both modern science and medicine is a myth. The church was least interested in science; in fact it stifled or tried to destroy free scientific inquiry. Only the hierarchy of the church was allowed education, which was discouraged or even denied to the general public. Any deviation from the fixed dogmas and notions of the Christian faith and church was punished as heresy.

During the outbreak of the Black Death in 1300, people turned to the church rather than to medicine. The church banned what little there was of Greek and Roman medicine to fight the plague, considering it heresy. After the plague, the church banned any formal discipline of medicine.

When Christianity ruled Europe in the Dark Ages, scientific and engineering advance ceased. The Roman aqueducts formed a stupendous engineering feat supplying clean water to citizens for centuries, a basic requirement to preserve health and prevent disease. When Christianity ruled Rome, the church no longer supported this great public service. The aqueducts became ruins—just a monument to the past glory of Rome. Christianity banned Roman Bath Houses and the ancient sewers no longer worked. This surely must have contributed to filth and disease.

The claim that Christianity established the first hospital is also incorrect. The earliest mention of cure centres came from Egyptians who aimed to provide medical care in their temples. Aesculapian temples in Greece that served the sick have already been mentioned. In India, King Ashoka founded hospitals providing both physicians and nursing staff in 230 BC. The Romans created Valetudiana for the care of sick slaves, gladiators and soldiers around 100 BC. The Sri Lankans are credited by some to be responsible for the first dedicated hospital (Sivkasotthi-Sala).

The church often proclaimed that it encouraged learning. It preserved to a significant extent the learning of past ages in its monasteries but it did not further or encourage either science or medicine. In fact the great universities of the West were founded after AD 1000—Salerno, Bologna, Montpellier, Salamanca, Padua, Sorbonne, Oxford and Cambridge flourished because they freed themselves from the influence and dictates of the Christian church. This is not to deny the fact that there were a number of scholars and physicians who were clerics within the fold of the church. Yet the diktat of Christianity ran counter to scientific inquiry or research. Centres of learning were established in the Middle East and Asia well before those in the West. Thus, the first teaching centre in the Middle

East for all faculties, including Medicine was founded by King Shapur of the Sassanian dynasty of Persia at Gundhishapur in the sixth and seventh centuries AD. This centre of learning in the Persian Empire was enriched by Nestorians (of the Nestorian faith), evicted by the Byzantine church, and was ultimately populated by scholars from all over the world. It is presumed to have the first teaching hospital of the world. In India, Taxila became one of the greatest centres of learning from the sixth century BC onwards. Nalanda, another great university town flourished from the fifth to the twelfth century AD. Benaras, also in India, was as ancient as Taxila and Nalanda. In fact it is the oldest surviving university in the world.

We need now to interrupt this discussion on religion and its relation to medicine in the West and take a fleeting glimpse at what transpired in two-thirds of the remaining world. Eastern culture, life and living continue to be permeated even today by a strong spiritualism and deep-rooted religious beliefs. In India, the ancient system of medicine is Ayurveda (the knowledge of longevity). Zysk has provided evidence to suggest that Ayurveda as a system of medicine has its roots in the ascetic milieu of Buddhism that prevailed in India in the fifth and sixth century BC. It is however possible that the birth of Ayurveda extends even further back into history, though concrete evidence to prove this may not be forthcoming. It is in fact more than likely that the roots of Ayurveda and its early sproutings were passed on by numerous gurus to their chelas (disciples) through word of mouth. Conceivably these little trickles of the ancient science of Ayurveda gathered through oral tradition became visible streams in the Buddhist period, joining together to culminate around the second century AD into the great treatises of *Charaka Samhita* and *Susruta Samhita*—Charaka being the great physician and Susruta, the great surgeon, both on par with Hippocrates of Greek fame. These medical treatises combine scientific and empiric medicine and surgery coloured by traditions and beliefs of that ancient era. Though religion did not hinder these compilations, there is little doubt that the thoughts, philosophy and religious beliefs embodied in the religious cum philosophical writings of the Vedas (1500 BC) must have formed the background that influenced Ayurvedic medicine.

Ayurveda continues to be practised in India today, particularly in many villages of this country comprising close to 70 per cent of a population of a billion. Till 1700, there was nothing to choose between Indian medicine (Ayurveda) and Western medicine. It was only later when discoveries in the natural sciences in the West fuelled far-reaching advances in Western medicine and surgery that medicine in India, China and the far East lagged behind.

In Africa, vast areas untouched or barely touched by civilizing forces still practise magic-cum-religious medicine, combined with some degree of empiricism. However, even areas of Africa which have been Christianized retain a deep sense of spirituality that partakes of the healing process. I have no personal experience of African medicine or the nature of African spirituality which influences medical beliefs. Jean Masanta Mapora identifies three basic elements of African spirituality—

1. Sacredness of life which should be preserved and respected as God's gift.
2. The relationship between illness, misfortune and sin. Sin is not taken in the usual biblical sense, but is associated with violation against taboos, disrespect for ancestors. Illness or misfortunes are related to personal or community transgressions.
3. The spirits of ancestors in African life is a part of African spirituality. 'African spirituality presents itself as an expression of the African soul.'

What is striking in the African approach is that healing is a community affair, in contrast to the individualistic approach of Western medicine. A sharing and caring community is necessary in the practice of African medicine.

Let us return to follow the further progress of Western medicine. The tree of medicine in the West has several roots. We have briefly discussed Greece and the school of rational medicine as also the Christian tradition. The third root is Arab-Islamic medicine, followed by the Renaissance and the European Enlightenment.

Arab-Islamic Medicine

The Arab-Islamic school had great physicians—Rhazes (al Rhazes), Avicenna (Ibn Sina) and Averroes (Ibn Rushid). The Greco-Roman works in medicine were translated into Arabic and Avicenna's magnum opus the five-volume *Canon of Medicine* was a standard work for six centuries. The Arab-Islamic school served as a cultural bridge between the Greco-Roman age and the Renaissance. Works of the former age translated into Arabic were thereby preserved and were retranslated into Latin in later centuries. This preservation would never have been possible without the advent of the religion of Islam and the Arab-Islamic scholars.

The Renaissance

The Renaissance was a throwback to the classical age of Greece and Rome. It was characterized by a process of rationalization and the freeing of man to an ever increasing extent from the shackles of religion and religious dogma. Andreas Vesalius, the great rebel of the Renaissance, founded modern anatomy with the publication of his great work *Di Humanis Corporis Fabrica*. This ushered in the medical Renaissance heralding the first step towards modern medicine. The Renaissance was an era of a scientific revolution of which medicine was an integral part.

The European Enlightenment

The process of rationalization of all sciences including medicine found optimal conditions for growth. Religion during this period and following this period right up to our present decade began to be gradually displaced or reduced in its importance. We have thus entered the modern and the post-modern age with a hope towards an increasingly secular culture, secular values and for better or worse secular medicine.

The above discussion brings into relief the growth of Western medicine from Greco-Roman times to the threshold of the future or post-modern era. It deals with the gradual secularization and rationalization of medicine. This has not been possible without struggle, with regard to the actual science of Western medicine. Christianity (both Catholicism and Protestantism), as expected, has opposed scientific discoveries that did not approximate or ran counter to teachings of the Gospel. Scientific facts do not stem from religious beliefs; it is religion which over the centuries that has had to yield to science. Yet, it was not until as late as 1993 that Pope John Paul II acquitted Galileo—360 years after his indictment for heresy—an indictment occasioned by his scientific belief that it was the earth that moved round the sun, and not the sun that moved round the earth. The Pope even conceded to the idea of evolution as 'an effectively proven fact'—130 years after Darwin first published his work. This enlightenment in the Christian religions should continue, as it should in all other religions, if science and religion were to stop being antagonistic to each other. I hold no brief for religious dogma, but I would separate religion and religious dogma from the innate spirituality of man, in which I firmly believe. The great prophets of the world—Zarathustra, Christ, Buddha, Mahavir did not preach religious dogma; they preached love, taught that the kingdom of Heaven was within each one of us, and spoke of the innate spirituality within man. If religion in its own way helps to nourish this innate spirituality, it is welcome.

I have used the word secularization earlier. Secularization is defined as a process of freeing or emancipation from religious constraints. It includes the rationalization of medicine according to proven scientific thoughts and concepts. Thus Western medicine has drifted away from healing systems that still hold humoral theories as in southeast Asia, the Arab world and Mexico. It has also drifted away from the theory of the 'meridians' within the body prevalent in China.

Some authors have introduced the concept of 'secularism' as the negative side of 'secularization.' Neubign used secularism to refer to a system of beliefs or an attitude which in principle denies the existence or significance of realities other than those which can be measured by the methods of modern science. Gerard Jensen (2008) in his paper on Western medicine—Secularised and Secularising, maintains 'it is this shadow side of secularism which concerns the evolution of a reductionistic biomedicine.'

Secularization of Western Medicine in Non-Western Countries

Western medicine began to penetrate non-Western countries when Vasco Da Gama set foot on the western coast of India. The spread of colonies into the poor non-Western world brought with it Western mores, attitudes, culture and also Western medicine. The latter was partly governmental, originating from colonial rule, but also to an extent from missionary work—Christian missions that accompanied or followed colonial penetration. These 'missions' had two functions —proselytizing and offering medical relief to local inhabitants within their domain and influence. Thus began the secularization of Western medicine in the remaining two-thirds of the world. It continues even after the emancipation and independence of all these various colonies. The introduction of Western medicine did not occur in a cultural vacuum. The local populations of each colony had their own ideas of illnesses and their approach to healing. The ancient art and science of Ayurveda in India and the spiritual aspect associated with African medicine have already been commented upon earlier. Even today far more of the one billion population of India practise Ayurveda as compared to Western medicine. And of those who practise Western medicine, many still consider that 'healing' has a spiritual aspect divorced from the science of medicine. Each traditional society whether in India, the Far East, China, Middle East, Africa, South America, or other societies scattered in islands or in other parts of the non-Western world has its own beliefs on medicine and healing. Religion, magic ritual, singly or in combination still hold sway in many primitive societies. These beliefs are bound to be gradually eroded to a varying extent with the spread of secular beliefs and the further secularization of Western medicine in the non-Western world. This secularization will be favoured by an increasingly tight-knit world, by free commerce and increasing trade, by the lure of consumerism, improving economies and better living standards. It will also be helped immensely by the burst in information technology over the last three decades. To what extent will the secularizing force of medicine succeed when it comes into contact and confrontation with cultures, beliefs and medical traditions quite distinct and different from the present Western world? It will never be able to oust completely the deep-rooted beliefs, customs, practices and cultures of different countries in the non-Western world. Its success will in fact be dependent on giving the different value systems of non-Western communities due consideration and respect; it will unquestionably also be aided and abetted to a very great extent by the dynamic process of acculturation, which may alter the foundations of traditional societies. Yet though traditional societies in the non-Western countries are bound to change, they will not resemble or closely approximate to the Western world. Spiritual beliefs and religion will colour both life and medicine to a lesser extent, but in the foreseeable future they can never be entirely abolished.

The post-modern age will have many relevant questions to debate. Can we negate with certainty the significance of realities other than those based on rationality emanating from science, or realities other than those which can be measured by the methods of natural science? I do not think so. As a practising physician who has lived for 50 years amidst death and disease, I feel that faith is a powerful and incalculable force that helps to heal. In the words of Osler, 'this powerful force can neither be weighed in a balance nor tested in a crucible in the laboratory.' Witness the thousands of the ailing and afflicted who make a pilgrimage to Lourdes and the documented instances where relief or perhaps even cure of suffering has been achieved. Think also of the millions over the world who have faith and claim relief after offering their respects to religious shrines in different parts of the world. Again, faith of a gravely ill patient in his or her doctor helps to heal. A critically ill patient has antennae (comparable to that of a child for his or her mother) that immediately latches on to the compassion shown by a truly caring doctor. The faith that this generates within the patient may well make the difference between life and death. Also, what is the value of prayer in medicine? I subscribe to the view—'More things are wrought by prayer than the world dreams of.' Prayer acts through increasing faith; it could be faith in God, in religion, faith in one's ancestors, faith in a new birth, in the permanence of life, in the indestructibility of the soul. Again it is often noted that those who think positively, who are optimistic, and think good thoughts get well faster when compared to those who have negative thoughts and feel they will never survive. Modern medicine will not accept the value of faith or prayer because neither faith nor prayer has the rationality emanating from science, nor can the effects of either be measured by the known methods of natural science. Unfortunately, the physician of the present era is focused on the science of curing, but has lost the art of healing.

Should secularized medicine in its present form be a shining, beckoning beacon for the remaining two-thirds of the world? I strongly doubt this. Western medicine which is an integral part of Western culture has brought in its wake numerous social, moral, ethical and cultural problems. I can only recommend to the reader Ivan Illich's treatise *Limits to Medicine*, wherein the author describes devastatingly the dangers of clinical iatrogenesis as also social and cultural iatrogenesis associated with present-day medicine. Ivan Illich unquestionably exaggerates and even distorts the hazards of Western medicine, but there is still an element of truth in his views.

Science, Medicine, God

The future holds the prospect of science and medicine questioning the need for religion and the existence of God. If human beings in the future are cloned as they almost certainly will be, science may well exclaim, 'Does God Exist?' Darwin's theory of evolution explains the genesis of man. After a delay at the stage of unicellular organism for billions of years, there commenced a slow evolution of increasingly complex living creatures culminating into the appearance of man on earth. Our evolutionary path has been for long unpredictable and beset by many hazards. Medical science claims that our evolutionary path was governed solely by chance and necessity. I believe this to be the apparent truth but not the whole truth. I believe that there is Providence or a Divine Force operating over and above and guiding the visible happenings of biological evolution. Evidence-based medicine (the proud slogan of contemporary medicine) would undoubtedly scoff at this unscientific, evidence-lacking concept. But then truth does not necessary cease to be so because it cannot be proven. On a lesser plane, this is applicable to some of the unpredictable and impossible to prove responses of man to disease and his unpredictable interaction with the art and science of medicine. On a higher plane this concept embraces some of the mysteries of the universe and of the existence of man as a conscious, thinking, experiencing, creating individual who comes into being at birth, but apparently ceases to be at death. It would be a profound tragedy for man and medicine if science were to refute the religious version of the universe or if scientific dogma were to negate the innate spirituality within man.

A Perspective on
Contemporary Medicine

*No one should approach the temple of science with the soul of
a money changer*

—Sir Thomas Brown

Over five thousand years of history, medicine evolved with
man—strengthened by observation, experience and judgement,
influenced by religion, faith, philosophy, economics, and enriched
above all by science. The advance of science and technology has been
stupendous. Over the last one hundred years, science has changed
the world and changed medicine with it. Immunology, genetics,
molecular biology which are the frontiers of contemporary medicine
owe their success largely to the advances in the natural sciences and
to technology.

Medicine and surgery are today capable of performing mind-
boggling feats deemed incredible half a century ago. Many a life
has been saved, many marvels performed, and many indeed must
have reaped the benefits from the knowledge and power that a
revolutionized medical science has to offer. Yet paradoxically, Man and
Medicine stand together on the threshold of the twenty-first century

sharing an uncertain future. There is a seething discontent against medicine and the medical profession among lay people, a discontent which is also shared by many within the profession. And why should this be so? The mechanization of medicine has robbed it of its essence, its humanism. All through the ages, from Imhotep, Hippocrates, Charaka, Susruta of antiquity, to Paré, Jenner, Hunter, Lister, Pasteur, Osler and several others, medicine meant care, compassion and a special empathy for the patient. Whatever garb medicine assumed, whatever philosophy it followed, whatever its blemishes and faults, human qualities lay entrenched at its very core, central to its being and existence. The essence of these human qualities expressed in a single word is humanity. Humanity is the sensibility which enables a physician to feel for the distress and suffering of a patient, prompting him to provide relief. True humanity in a physician is a fount of sympathy and care. The advent of machines, sophisticated gadgets and increasing technology has depersonalized medicine, lessened its humanity and adversely affected the doctor-patient relationship. Patients today are often made to relate to machines than to human beings and doctors relate more to sophisticated gadgetry than to patients.

A companion-in-arms of increasing mechanization is increasing superspecialization. A superspecialist is of unquestionable importance in certain well-defined situations and can be an invaluable asset to modern medicine. But an over-enthusiastic encouragement of superspecialities is self-defeating, for it negates the holistic aspect of medicine. Medicine cannot be compartmentalized. No organ functions in splendid isolation, for the human system is a mysterious yet integrated whole. A poorly trained, or self-proclaimed specialist (and there are many such in India), or the one who lacks the necessary background and experience in general medicine and surgery ignores this basic concept. He tends to view medicine with myopic eyes, loses his perspective and his sense of priorities and can thereby discredit medicine. Contemporary medicine often presents the tragic-comic scene of a critically ill individual being looked after by a number of superspecialists aided and abetted by the trappings of technology and science. Each specialist concentrates solely on his small exclusive field of expertise; the overall aspect of disease and of the patient as a human being suffering from disease is then easily lost.

To the mechanization of medicine is added the sin of commercialization. Money is increasingly a driving force in today's medicine. Its acquisition through the charging of unreasonable fees even from the poor and unaffording goes against its basic tenets. The healing art in many parts of the world is more a business than a profession. Even worse, it is a business that has become increasingly corrupt. What is more corrupt than the practice of doctors who on purpose refer unsuspecting, vulnerable patients from one specialist to another for no reason other than profit? Or what is more corrupt than the nefarious practice of commissions demanded by general practitioners from a specialist to whom a patient is referred? Corrupt practices such as these are commonplace in the larger cities of India and perhaps occur with varying frequency and in various guises in other parts of the world.

One other major drawback of contemporary medicine is its crippling expense in relation to investigations, treatment and the cost of hospitalization. This is partly due to the fact that the physician of today has forgotten the art of medicine and remains deeply immersed in its science. His rapport is with machines and not with patients; it is technology that dictates his course of action and not his clinical judgement. History-taking becomes a neglected art; he forgets to use his senses—his eyes, ears and hands, but remembers numbers, equations and formulae. Expensive investigations and expensive modes of treatment often result when simple tests and simpler measures would have easily sufficed.

In the West, the escalating cost of medicine has prompted the State or insurance companies to exert a control over its practice. This is unfortunate for several reasons. The control over medicine should come from within; it would hurt medicine if it is forced from without. In the poor countries of the world where the State has by and large abjured its responsibilities for patient care and where insurance for illnesses is meagre and unsatisfactory, the financial burden often falls directly on the patient and his relatives. This is a cruel burden that can reduce a family to penury and despair.

A seething antagonism against contemporary medicine has led both to increasing litigation against doctors and a search for relief through 'alternative medicine'. Homeopathy, Ayurvedic medicine, acupuncture, herbal and folk medicine, spiritual healing, a new form of the 'laying of hands' called Reiki, all have an increasing demand today. Special centres both in the West and the East have been set up to scientifically assess the values of some of these alternative methods of medicine. The modern physician in his love for science and technology has forgotten to appreciate that faith and nature are two of the greatest healing forces that can mend and restore the mind and body. He also needs to be reminded that ancient systems of medicine like Ayurveda, herbal and folk medicine have stood the test of time and are still effectively used by millions all over the world.

Institutionalized medicine has also contributed to malpractice. It is a matter of prestige for every hospital in the poorer countries of the world to be equipped with the latest in Western technology and science. Yet rapid advances in medicine render most machines obsolete within five to at the most ten years. If an institution or hospital is to profit after spending a fortune on machines, it has to feed the machines. Patients become the fodder for these machines. If an audit were carried out on the cost-effectiveness of modern-day investigations in medicine, the result would be shocking.

Perhaps the underlying explanation for the decline in the ethics of contemporary medicine is a change in the sense of values in our world. A burning desire for material gain and wealth at any cost dominates life today. It is indeed difficult for any profession to remain as an island of high-mindedness and virtue when surrounded by a sea of filth and corruption. The island is first eroded and then swamped. But the medical profession has an ancient heritage to cherish and maintain. This is being slowly but increasingly realized all over the world and there is now a growing force imbued with a determination to uproot the canker eating into the heart of medicine.

Let us now examine the content of contemporary medicine. To an extent, it can claim credit for the control, eradication or near-extinction of many infectious diseases that prevailed at the outset of the Industrial Age in the West. Plague, cholera, smallpox, diphtheria, typhoid, tetanus, scarlet fever, measles, whooping cough, poliomyelitis are some of the scourges that are rarely encountered or have been rendered more or less extinct. Yet victory over these diseases in the West has been more through effective preventive measures rather than through drugs, or the use of sophisticated gadgetry and technology. It is clean drinking water, good nutrition, improved housing, sanitation, hygiene, education and thriving economies that have led to the conquest of many infectious diseases. Man was on the road to the conquest of age-old infections well before modern technology captured medicine. Perhaps the greatest gift of medicine to mankind is the discovery of vaccines to prevent disease. Outstanding among these discoveries is that of Edward Jenner in the prevention of smallpox.

It is of interest that tuberculosis was as much a scourge in Europe and the United States in the nineteenth century as it is in India and other poor countries of the world today. Modern anti-TB drugs are effective and have reduced the incidence and mortality of TB. But the maximum decline in the disease occurred well before the introduction of anti-TB drugs and even well before the first sanitarium opened to isolate patients with tuberculosis. That drugs alone are not enough is seen in the increasing incidence, morbidity and mortality of tuberculosis in India and Africa. These countries can never wipe out tuberculosis and numerous other infections without an improvement in their economies, their public health and education.

The above discussion should not detract from the merit of newly discovered drugs, effective antibiotics and the use of various medical and surgical procedures that have saved human lives which would otherwise have been surely lost. Acute meningitis, infections of heart valves, acute septicaemia from fulminant organisms are just a few examples of diseases which had a universal mortality till the discoveries of modern medicine came into use. Advances in surgery over the last 50 years have indeed been even more enthralling. Today the surgeon can 'touch' almost every nook and corner of the human anatomy to achieve what he sets out to do. Surgery on the heart for congenital and acquired heart disease, coronary artery bypass surgery, thoracic surgery, neurosurgery, plastic surgery, cancer surgery, and surgical advances in all other specialties are landmarks that evoke unstinted praise and admiration. Laparoscopic surgery popularly called 'key-hole' surgery is a triumph of technology and surgical skill; it has markedly reduced postoperative pain, postoperative complications and the duration of hospital stay. Hip replacement (hip arthroplasty), knee replacement (knee arthroplasty), shoulder replacement, replacement of other joints by the use of prosthetic implants have relieved crippling pain and disability caused most commonly by osteoarthritis but by other arthritides as well.

It would be impossible to dwell at length on the numerous advances that have brought great benefits to mankind. I wish, however, to briefly describe just one of these advances in surgery—the surgery of organ transplantation. I do so for the following reasons. First, this advance is the culmination of joint efforts of science, technology and surgical skill—a combination that is the hallmark of most advances in contemporary medicine and surgery. Secondly, though organ transplant surgery is a phenomenal advance, it has brought in its wake, particularly in poor developing countries such as India, difficult, murky ethical issues. It is therefore a perfect illustration of the bright and dark side of contemporary medicine. Thirdly, the earlier part of this essay as also the final portion that is to follow, focuses on some of the disadvantages of contemporary medicine. For a balanced perspective, I needs must dwell for a while on at least one of the many benefits that contemporary medicine has to offer. Finally, the surgical advances in organ transplantation are perhaps the most dramatized, receiving a great deal of media coverage and exercising a great fascination for the lay public. The operative skills for human allotransplantation (an allograft is a transplanted organ or tissue from a genetically non-identical member of the same species) were present long before the requirements for the postoperative survival of the graft were discovered. The idea that organ transplants were feasible must have occurred to man several centuries ago, for history is replete with apocryphal accounts of transplants in an age when science was well-nigh non-existent. We read of the Chinese physician Pien Chiao who reportedly exchanged hearts between a man of strong spirit but weak will with one of a man with a weak spirit but strong will in order to achieve a balanced harmony in each.

The Roman Catholic Church gives an account of the third-century saints Damian and Cosmas replacing the gangrenous leg of the Roman Justinian with the leg of a recently deceased Ethiopian. Justinian was said to have survived with one lower limb black and the other white! If we graduate from miracles to facts then the first skin transplantation could be attributed to the great Indian surgeon Susruta in the second century BC. He used an autografted skin transplant in nose reconstruction (rhinoplasty). Many centuries later an Italian surgeon Gaspare Tagliacozzi performed successful skin autografts. He failed consistently when he used allografts suggesting for the first time the possibility of rejection of the allograft long before the mechanism of rejection was clearly understood.

The history of organ transplant surgery for many centuries was a litany of disaster till about the middle of the twentieth century. It was Peter Medawar working for the National Institute of Medical Research in the UK who first threw light on the nature of immune mechanisms responsible for rejection of allografts. He advocated the use of immunosuppressive drugs to counter rejection. The first drug to be used was cortisone, followed by azathioprine. However, it was only after the discovery of cyclosporine in 1970 that surgeons had a powerful immunosuppressive agent. Organ transplants now became a refreshing reality. Kidney transplants for those in irreversible renal failure became increasingly successful and changed the lives of thousands from abject misery and certain death to a life of reasonable good health and productivity. Immunosuppressants, however, prevented rejection of a transplanted organ or tissue yet promoted infection through suppression of normal immune responses. This is a danger that persists to the present day.

Perhaps the most dramatic of all organ transplants is the heart transplant. The first successful heart transplant was performed on 3 December 1967 by Christiaan Barnard in Cape Town, South Africa and Louis Washkansky, the recipient survived for 18 days. The event was to my mind spoilt by a circus of publicity distasteful in the extreme. There followed a spate of heart transplants at Stanford University Hospital and at the Texas Heart Institute at Houston, Texas, as also in prominent European centres. Survival rates were low with most patients dying within six months. By 1984, two-thirds of all transplant patients survived for five years or more. Today a number of these transplants have survived 10 years.

Heart transplants were followed by successful lung transplants, heart and lung transplants as also transplants of other organs and tissues. The success rate of transplant surgery both as a result of improved technique and more effective immunosuppression has increased in the last 20 years. The critical issue is the limitation imposed by the scarcity of sufficient donor organs. Cadaveric organs are difficult to obtain in some countries like India, but living donor transplants are coming into greater use with regard to both liver and kidney transplant surgery. Surgeons are now moving into more risky fields, trying out multiple organ transplants in humans as also whole-body transplant research in animals.

Advances in immunosuppression are also keeping apace—both with regard to preventing rejection of the transplanted organ and minimizing as far as possible the complications of infection related to immunosuppression. Thus researchers have been looking into steroid-free immunosuppression to avoid the side-effects of steroids. Also, Calcineurin-Inhibitor-Free Immunosuppression is currently undergoing extensive trials. If successful it could allow sufficient immunosuppression with regimes that include calcineurin inhibitors without producing effects like nephrotoxicity. Ideally, researchers are aiming at a regime which prevents rejection of the transplanted organ or tissue and yet minimizes the risk of complicating infection. But this is a trespass into the future!

Besides the kidney, liver, heart, lung, heart-lung, other organs and tissues successfully transplanted include the pancreas, intestine, the hand, cornea, skin graft including facial replant (autograft) and extremely rarely a face transplant, islets of Langerhans, penis, bone marrow/adult stem cell, blood vessels, heart valve (porcine / bovine xenograft), bone and skin.

Transplant surgery has unfortunately brought in its wake several ethical problems. The most criminal of these is the sale of organs, particularly the kidney from the poor who are prepared to donate a kidney in exchange for money. This practice still exists in poor countries including India, in spite of the most stringent laws against this heinous crime. It is a crying shame on the doctors who participate in this traffic as also on those within and outside the medical profession who quietly acquiesce to it.

In spite of the advances of contemporary medicine, the world today and the West in particular, face the 'modern epidemics' of coronary heart disease, chronic bronchitis, hypertension, cancer, diabetes, mental disorders and several other diseases and disabilities. Medicine does not know why many of these diseases occur; it offers relief but has no cure. Contemporary medicine has also no satisfactory answer to the occurrence of deadly new infections such as AIDS, or the deadly haemorrhagic viral infections fortunately localized to a few regions of the world. It has also to contend with the recrudescence of old infections, such as tuberculosis and malaria.

The progress of medicine from ancient times to the present era is evident; yet there is a 'seamier' side to this progress which has been eloquently stressed by Ivan Illich in his book *Limits to Medicine*. Illich contends that the medical establishment has become a major threat to health. To my mind, this is an overstatement, an exaggeration that is a travesty of truth. Yet his contention that the 'medicalization of life' has three major disadvantages does carry a germ of truth within it and needs careful consideration.

The first disadvantage is the production of 'clinical iatrogenesis' ('iatros' in Greek means 'physician'; 'genesis' means 'to make'). Iatrogenic diseases in medicine are those produced by physicians either through treatment or investigations, or by hospitals in which patients are treated. But then iatrogenic disease is as old as medicine. It has been an inseparable companion of medicine since antiquity. The pharmacopoeias up to the nineteenth century contained substances which must have done far more harm than good. To give just one example, the frequent practice of blood-letting which persisted up to the early years of the twentieth century, almost always hastened a patient's demise. The only excuse for iatrogenic disease in the earlier ages is that medicine then did not know and was none the wiser that it could inflict harm. But today we do know the potential iatrogenesis of medicine. Unfortunately, our awareness has not helped.

Contemporary medicine has indeed produced an epidemic of iatrogenesis, because the more potent the drug, the more sophisticated the gadgetry and the more invasive the procedures used in diagnosis or management, the greater the risk of harm to patients. Yet it will be impossible in the foreseeable future to separate the art and science of medicine completely from iatrogenesis. There is no drug worth its name which is totally free of side-effects. Also, dreadful illnesses often demand risky procedures or potent drugs with inherent toxicity to the human system. The practice of medicine forces a physician to take a balanced risk if a critically ill patient is to be salvaged. It is not just a knowledge of the science of medicine that determines this risk; it is also determined by experience, judgement and wisdom—it involves in equal measure the art that constitutes medicine even today.

The second disadvantage of contemporary medicine is the production of 'social iatrogenesis'– by which is meant the creation of an environment which no longer has the ability to allow people in society to look after themselves. People are thus hopelessly dependent on the medical system and the medical system functions in a manner to ensure that this remains so. The medicalization of life would prompt people to consume medicine, seek hospitalization or medical treatment for inadequate reasons. An encouragement to take recourse to institutionalized medicine perpetuates the stranglehold of the medical profession and medical institutions over society. Contemporary medicine has also insinuated itself into the health consciousness of people through powerful media coverage, aided and abetted by the internet. It is the 'Big Brother' warning you of the hidden hazards in daily life, instructing you what to eat and what not to eat, what to do and what not to do, how to live and how not to live. Some of the offered advice is sensible, but some amounts to quackery. An obsession with preserving health has led to an anxiety amounting to a neurosis, breeding what James Le Fanu calls 'the worried well'. The well are worried sick because of medical experts warning them of the hidden dangers to health!

Almost certainly the excessive dependence of society on institutionalized medicine is a passing phase and will be tempered by better judgement and by an increasing awareness of the need for a healthier relationship between the two. It must be remembered that the link between man and medicine is impossible to sever. Both are dependent on each other; it is important that neither takes advantage of the other.

The third disadvantage of contemporary medicine according to Illich is the encouragement of a cultural iatrogenesis. This it effectively does by sapping the will of the people to suffer their reality. Suffering is a realistic human response. Pain and suffering are as much a part of life and living as joy and pleasure. Illich claims that the term 'suffering' has become almost useless for designating a realistic human response, because it evokes superstition, sadomasochism or the rich man's condescension for the lot of the poor. Our world has different cultures and each culture has evolved over centuries its own *gestalt* of health and disease. Eastern cultures, notably Hindu and Buddhist cultures regard the vicissitudes of life, as also 'suffering' in any form, with a certain degree of acceptance, fortitude and philosophy. I do not for a moment believe that one should 'suffer' merely for the sake of 'suffering' or 'suffer' merely to experience the realistic human response. Pain and suffering can and should be relieved, but Medicine should realize that they cannot be totally obliterated, or wiped off the surface of the earth. It is impossible to do so, just as it is impossible to fight the inevitability of death. Illich believes that institutionalized medicine's war against 'suffering' and also its resolve to fight and ward off death to the bitter end constitute cultural iatrogenesis. 'This domineering moral enterprise has undermined the ability of individuals to face their own reality, to express their own values and to accept the inevitable and often irremediable pain and impairment, decline and death.' In fact, the medicalization of pain, suffering, dying and even death is an attempt to do for people what their culture and heritage has equipped them to do for themselves. This will increasingly benefit medicine, but after a point will cease to benefit man. There is some truth in Illich's diatribe against contemporary medicine but it is not the whole truth. He has given us the dark side of the picture, just as there are many who only see the bright side of the picture. The truth lies in-between.

The attitudes of contemporary medicine require a change, yet it must be remembered that it is society which has conditioned some of these attitudes. A great deal more is expected of medicine today than it can offer. The stupendous advances in medical science, the glamour and excitement of so-called miracle cures flashed across the world by the information media, have led people to believe that contemporary medicine is all-knowing, all-powerful and all-successful. This is unfortunately far from the truth. *There are limits to medicine— today and in the foreseeable future.* As has been already mentioned earlier, if one takes the sum total of all diseases, there are just a few that medicine can completely cure, though there are many that it can alleviate. Therefore the great expectations from medicine are at times unreal and often unfulfilled. When people experience this fact personally and also encounter the unseemly aspects of medicine with its escalating costs, it arouses disappointment, distrust and anger. The doctor-patient relationship which is the essence of medicine stands inevitably poisoned.

The decline of values today is not restricted to medicine and the medical profession. It afflicts all professions and the whole of society, perhaps even to a greater extent than that observed in medicine. The frustration of patients and relatives is often translated into litigation and a demand for compensation. Not uncommonly this demand is motivated by a greed for money than by a true sense of injured justice. To protect himself the doctor falls back on defensive medicine. He over-investigates to ensure that he is not sued for missing out on rare disorders, he uses the more powerful weapons of medicine and science involving greater risks of iatrogenicity when simpler ones would have sufficed. When faced with a life-threatening emergency he would rather let the patient die than take the risk of doing a procedure or offering treatment, which though inherently risky constitutes the only hope to salvage life. He progressively divorces himself from all that really matters in medicine. This is no excuse for malpractice, incompetency, callousness, disregard for patient welfare, even in the presence of utmost provocation. These are infirmities, pockmarks that need to be wiped off the face of medicine. Yet it must be admitted that a healthy interaction and interrelation between medicine and society is a reciprocal affair. Both need to look at each other with fresh eyes, both need to communicate with each other if this indeed is to transpire.

In most countries of the world disputes between doctors and patients are decided by duly constituted professional bodies or by courts of law. In India the doctor is more often brought before a 'consumer court' for any alleged incompetence or offence. This is because the highest court of justice in the country has decreed that the practice of medicine is similar to a consumer industry and the service rendered by a doctor to a patient is akin to a 'consumer product'. Nothing in my opinion could be further from the truth. It is patently absurd to equate the years of study, the knowledge, expertise, experience, wisdom and above all the care lavished on a patient with a 'consumer product'. The doubts, anxieties, uncertainties, the sleepless nights, the anguish that goes into an irrevocable life or death decision are surely different from the gift-wrap paper and the consumer product enclosed within, however expensive this product may be. After all, is it not the human values of good medicine that distinguish it from a business or industry?

Sadly, the reason for this predicament at least in India lies chiefly with the medical profession. The crisis has arisen because of the attitudinal changes in modern-day medicine described earlier. It has been further accentuated by a lack of internal audit within the profession. The medical bodies that should adjudicate and mete out justice to both patients and doctors are seen by many to have not lived up to their responsibilities. Lacking internal control, a control is sought to be established from without. But in doing so, the courts in India have done a disservice to the profession and in the long run to society whose rights they are keen to protect. Their decision has lent legal sanctity to the concept of medicine being considered a business and the service of a doctor being akin to a consumer product. It has only served to freeze and perpetuate the unsatisfactory state of affairs and not improve them.

Contemporary medicine faces a special challenge in India and other third world countries as health problems in these countries are significantly different from those in the West. Infection and infectious diseases (with the sole exception of smallpox) are still as prevalent in these poor countries as they were in the West more than a hundred years ago. Poor nutrition and poverty form the backdrop against which many common diseases unfold. Unfortunately, India has the dubious distinction of also facing the 'new epidemics' prevalent today in the West—coronary heart disease, chronic bronchitis, cancer, diabetes to name just a few. It is not that science and technology incorporated in contemporary Western medicine should be abandoned in the poor countries of the world. Their use must be viewed in a balanced perspective. Much greater attention must be paid to the preventive aspects of medicine. Far more money should be allocated to providing clean water, good nutrition, sanitation, housing, education, population control and the use of preventive vaccines, than to the purchase of glittering machines and to the building of five-star hospitals in the urban centres of these countries. Medical education in a country such as India should be oriented to problems facing this country and not to those facing the West. Ethics should be taught more by example and precept than by oft-repeated platitudes. An equitable distribution of meagre resources with a focussed attention on problems afflicting 70 per cent of the population residing in the villages of India may well be rewarded by greater benefits to greater numbers of people.

Implementation of health measures in poor countries does not require the adoption of expensive Western methods of health delivery. Villagers locally recruited and trained have been shown to impart basic healthcare efficiently and at an infinitely smaller cost. A growing economy, increasing education, honest, efficient governance and self-reliance are the basic necessities that can effectively curb disease and promote healthcare in the poor countries of the world.

In conclusion, contemporary medicine reflects the virtues and shortcomings, the strength and weakness of our contemporary world.

From an overall perspective, medicine today has benefited mankind more than ever before. Those who mock it and see no good within it are often the first to seek its protection when the need arises. It is sheer cant and bigotry to believe with Ivan Illich that the medical establishment is a hazard to health. Even so, we must recognize and admit its faults and blemishes. The crisis in contemporary medicine is paradoxically related to the crisis caused by over-rapid progress, and to shattered expectations. Its basic drawback stems from the overpowering dominance of its science which has robbed it of its humanity and submerged its art. Science divorced from humanity and art, science which is allowed to dictate and command rather than to serve and obey will be a tragedy for both medicine and man. The medicine of today and the future must recognize this fact. Contemporary medicine needs to recapture its spirit of humanism and to re-establish the special empathy in a doctor-patient relationship if it is to restore its pristine image and regain the universal respect and approval of man. It can only do so if it divorces itself from the lure of money, raises its ethical standards and places the welfare and care of patients above all else.

Medicine in the Future

The longer you look back, the further you look forward.
—WINSTON CHURCHILL

The future is already upon us. The writing is on the wall; it is there for all to see. Medical science will battle in the twenty-first century to discover the secret of our origin and the mystery of our mortality. The twenty-first century will be the century of biotechnology—genetics, molecular and reproductive biology will dominate research in medicine and strongly influence its practice. The quantum leap in our knowledge of biogenetics and reproductive biology has given us the incredible power to control the destiny of the human species and the potential to shape and direct our future evolutionary path. This would have appeared unthinkable a few years ago but is nevertheless very true today.

The seeds of future research in these fields were planted in 1953 when Watson and Crick unravelled the detailed structure and the self-copying code of the DNA molecule. For those unfamiliar with biology or medicine a brief explanation of what medical science has achieved and continues to achieve is necessary. The human body contains 75 trillion cells. The nucleus of each cell contains 46 chromosomes arranged in 23 pairs. Each chromosome is a wadded-up strand of DNA. Unfolded and stretched the DNA strand would measure about three to nine feet in length and 20 atoms across. Genes are segments of DNA that contain the instructions to make proteins— the building blocks of life. The DNA molecule has hundreds of millions of base-pairs. The sum of the DNA in all 46 chromosomes is the human genome. The Human Genome Project was initiated in 1990 with the objective to determine the complete sequence of the human genome. The project was successfully completed in 2000, five years before the projected date of completion. The science of medicine has now an access to the book of life—the precise biochemical code of each of these genes which by and large determine every physical characteristic within the human body.

The Impact of Genomic Science on Disease

Genomic science in the near future should then determine how each gene functions and more importantly how a malfunctioning gene can produce or influence specific disease. A number of diseases are genetic in origin while others have a genetic component. If a gene responsible for a disease is once localized and mapped it can be cloned through bioengineering techniques. The future potential for medicine is immense. The disease-producing cloned gene could be used for diagnostic purposes and this in some instances could initiate preventive strategies. An example is the indication for colonoscopy in individuals at genetically high risk for colonic cancer. The cloned disease-producing gene could also enable us to understand the basic biological defect in the disease. Genes sometimes produce proteins linked to the disease. Researchers call these genes and proteins 'targets'. Drugs could target the gene or target the abnormal disease-related protein produced by the gene, thereby altering its action. Finally, medical science is heading towards the future prospect of effective gene therapy. An abnormal gene responsible for a particular malfunction or disease could theoretically be countered by introducing into the body or the organ involved the appropriate normal functioning gene. This would restore normal function and thereby reverse disease.

The theoretical potential of the science of genetics to aid medicine in the amelioration and conquest of disease in the future is unquestioned. Admittedly, as yet this has not come about. The question therefore arises—will the future see this happen? Will the science of genetics benefit man and medicine in the future, or will it end as an expensive futile journey down a blind alley? In my opinion genetic science has made fundamental discoveries that almost certainly will come of use in time to come. There has often been a delay of several decades before great discoveries in natural sciences have been put to use for the benefit of mankind. The diagnostic consequences of gene discovery (prediction of susceptibility to disease) will almost certainly be available in the near future, though the interaction between one or more genes and the environment in producing a specific disease may be difficult to interpret. The time sequence of simple and cost-effective curative therapies (either drugs or gene therapy) is unpredictable and may take several decades.

Future medicine will attempt to contain the 'new epidemics' of cancer, hypertension, diabetes, coronary heart disease, cerebrovascular disease, chronic bronchitis, mental disorders, and disorders affecting an increasingly ageing population. There is no true cure visible on the horizon for any of these afflictions. Cancer will continue to have the maximum funding for research. Molecular pathology may perhaps revolutionize the diagnosis and treatment of cancer. A tumour's molecular fingerprints will determine how it behaves. Most researchers believe that the future holds no single magic bullet against cancer, because 'there are probably a million cancers, maybe as there are patients with cancers'. However, emerging research from molecular pathology laboratories holds out a promise for specific tools for early detection, and for choosing treatment that is far more appropriate in a given situation than exists today. The identification of genes that can induce the synthesis of growth-control molecules has stimulated a search for specific anticancer drugs that can change the activity of selected genes so that the synthesis of RNA from a DNA template is selectively inhibited.

The future also holds promise in its ability to modify the genetic basis of immunity—the technique of immunomodulation. When genes controlling the synthesis of cytokines are introduced into cancer cells and lymphocytes, they trigger a cytotoxic response that results in death of the cancer cells and other diseased cells. Unfortunately, cytokines are not sufficiently selective and cause unwanted side-effects through damage and death of healthy cells. Methods to improve selectivity include the use of chemically modified anticancer drugs which remain nontoxic till they reach their target site. Once in place they are activated by light (photoactivation), or by monoclonal antibodies exerting a selective distinctive action on cancer cells.

Monoclonal antibodies unfortunately have not lived up to expectations. Even so, the theoretical concept underlying their use is attractive and research on their therapeutic application is certain to continue. A possible future for monoclonal antibodies is in the treatment of multiple sclerosis, an autoimmune disease in which the lymphocytes instead of performing their usual protective role attack and injure the brain and spinal cord. Research is being directed to finding the appropriate monoclonal antibodies that latch on to a feature of lymphocytes that will prevent them from injuring the central nervous system. This is not beyond the realm of possibility. Scientists are also attempting to attach drugs to monoclonal antibodies to ensure that the drugs exactly reach the desired target thereby producing the expected results with little or no side-effects.

Genetic Science and the Future

Gene-based drug therapy, gene therapy and the increasing use of recombinant DNA vaccines in the prevention of disease are the obvious happy non-controversial benefits that should result from our increasing mastery over genetic science. However, the potential of genetic engineering and of advances in biotechnology could conceivably produce incredible revolutionary changes in mankind. These could include new sources of organs and tissues for transplants, methods to halt the ageing process, cloning of human beings, producing designer babies, and perhaps modifying the human genome in an attempt to improve upon the several million years of Darwinian selection.

Let us first briefly recapitulate what genetic science has achieved today so that we have a base that enables us to imagine the exciting yet terrifying future. It was in 1986 that the FDA approved the first genetically engineered Hepatitis B vaccine for use in humans. As mentioned earlier the International Human Genome Project was launched in 1990 under the leadership of James Watson. The three billion-dollar project which was to map and sequence all human DNA by 2003, was completed three years earlier—in the year 2000. The American geneticist W. French Anderson performed in 1990 the first gene therapy on a four-year-old girl afflicted with a congenital immune deficiency disease. American and British scientists in 1992 devised techniques to test human embryos for genetic defects such as cystic fibrosis and haemophilia. In 1993 researchers at George Washington University cloned human embryos and nurtured them in Petri dishes for several days drawing great criticism from many sources. The world stood astounded and a trifle aghast when on 27 February 1997 embryologist Ian Wilmut heading a research team at Scotland's Roslin Institute reported in *Nature* the cloning of a sheep named Dolly, from the cell of an adult ewe. This was followed in 1998 by researchers at Hawaii University cloning a mouse, creating dozens of copies and three generations of cloned clones. In Japan scientists at Kinki University have cloned eight identical calves from a single adult cow. The Oregon Regional Primate Research Centre in Beaverton, United States has reported the birth of two successfully cloned rhesus monkeys. The successful cloning of animals has sent shock waves throughout the world raising both ethical issues and moral dilemmas.

Research on the controlled development of embryonic stem cells also holds promise for the future. In the human being, the only time that cells possess the potential to develop into any or all body parts is in early pregnancy when stem cells have not begun to differentiate. In the autumn of 1998 scientists at the Wisconsin University finally managed to isolate embryonic stem cells and induced them to grow into neural, gut, muscle and bone cells. The research is in its infancy and may perhaps have its limitations. If, however, stem cell growth and differentiation into any desired tissue is achieved, medicine would be revolutionized. Doctors would be able to replace injured and dead tissues of disease with healthy tissue. Perhaps organs like the liver, heart and kidney could also be grown in the laboratory, making transplant surgery available to all.

Cloning holds a similar potential. As in the case of Dolly the sheep, cloning involves the use of a developed somatic cell and reactivating the genome within; so that its instruction to develop is reset to the earliest pristine state. Once this transpires the cell develops into a full-fledged animal genetically identical to the parent. The cloning technique used above is best termed the 'somatic cell nuclear transfer'. In Dolly's case the somatic cell was taken from the udder of an adult ewe; the nuclear transfer was effected by inserting the genomic material into an oocyte which had been earlier ennucleated i.e. had its nucleus removed.

As with the development of stem cells, cloning could in the future also help to develop organs for transplants or healthy tissues to replace diseased tissues. In the not too distant future organs and tissues for transplants may well be up for sale in the shopping centres of many large cities of the world. If animals can be cloned, the cloning of humans though technically more difficult will almost certainly one day come about. The emotional, ethical and legal problems that the future world would then face may well be insurmountable.

The frightening aspect of genetic science (at least to me) is the prospect of the possible results of the insertion of functional genetic material into the human germ cells—sperm or ovum. This could well change the course of our future evolution, could affect nature's process of natural selection and in the centuries or perhaps in the millennia to come create a new form of living species that would be unrecognizable to humans inhabiting the world today. Though no government wishes to take steps to initiate or sanction this research, the demand to move in the above direction in the years to come may be irresistible. Today in advanced centres of fertility and reproduction in the West, parents can choose a child's sex and screen for genetic illness. Gene therapy to correct genetic illness in embryos is, however, still a few years away. As yet, the genes responsible for most of the physical and mental attributes have not been identified. Perhaps in a decade or two these would be known so that it will be possible to screen embryos and foetuses for different physical and mental characteristics. If gene therapy lives up to its potential, parents may not only want undesirable traits of their unborn child weeded out, they would perhaps insist on inserting genes they desire. I shudder to think that the new millenium after some decades may well open into an era of 'designer babies'. The overall prospect is awesome and frightening. It may read as science fiction today, but we must remember that much of science fiction in the past has come to be true in the present. Will the future see medical science and technology change man into an unrecognizable species?

Infections of the Future

The poor countries of the world including India will continue to grapple against infections for several decades. The infections that will dominate the first decades of the present century in countries like India and Africa will be tuberculosis (TB) and AIDS. These two diseases will also continue to take a toll of human life in the West. India in particular is heading for an explosive increase in Human

Immunodeficiency Virus (HIV) infection. It is estimated that about 40 million Indians will be infected by HIV by the first two decades of the twenty-first century. Global statistics in 2008 show that 33 million people are infected with HIV of which two million are children under the age of 15 years. Total AIDS deaths in 2007 were two million. The danger from TB in developing countries is even worse. In 1993 the WHO declared TB as a 'global emergency'. In 1995 there were more deaths from TB than in any other year. The years 1990-99 saw 90 million new cases and close to 30 million deaths. There were an estimated 9.2 million new cases of TB in 2006 of which 0.7 million were HIV-positive. In the same year, there were an estimated 1.5 million deaths from TB in HIV-negative people and 0.2 million among people infected with HIV. This ancient disease is today the largest cause of death from a single pathogen. In the global context it is responsible for twice the number of deaths that are caused by AIDS, diarrhoea and all other parasitic diseases put together.

Tuberculosis and AIDS are companions-in-arms; they aid and abet each other. The increasing incidence of HIV infection and AIDS in many poor countries of the world will bring in its wake a six to tenfold increase in the incidence of tuberculosis. It has been aptly stated that 'TB has been a time bomb, AIDS has shortened its fuse'. Like the horsemen of the Apocalypse these two diseases promise a savage destruction of humanity in India and Africa in the twenty-first century. The problem in the future will be further compounded by the rising incidence of multiple drug-resistant (MDR) tuberculosis. Data on the incidence of MDR TB in India is sparse, but one large survey showed an incidence as high as 44%. If even half this incidence is representative of the country, it forecasts the death of many more millions in the first few decades of the twenty-first century. Reports show an estimated 0.5 million deaths from MDR TB in 2006 worldwide. Recent findings from a survey conducted by WHO and Centers for Disease Control and Prevention (CDC) on data from

2000-04 found that Extensive Resistant Tuberculosis (XDR TB, also referred to as Extreme Drug Resistance, is MDR TB that is also resistant to three or more of the six classes of second-line drugs) has been identified in all regions of the world but is most frequent in the countries of the former Soviet Union and in Asia. The WHO has advocated Directly Observed Therapy (DOTS) regime to help in the conquest of TB, pointing to its success in reducing very significantly the incidence of the disease and in preventing MDR TB in studies carried out in New York, Tanzania and China. But these are small studies carried out by motivated medical and social workers. It is impossible in my opinion to significantly alter the high incidence of TB and for that matter any other widely prevalent infection by drugs alone in a country such as India. The size of the country, the inaccessibility of so many areas within the country, the corruption, dishonesty and lack of motivation at all levels and above all the poverty, ignorance, overcrowding, lack of sanitation and hygiene coupled with poor nutrition are great impediments to the successful implementation of DOTS.

René Dubois in 1952 wrote: 'Tuberculosis is the ultimate social disease! A disease that medicine never cured, wealth never warded off'. The road to its conquest is the road to socioeconomic emancipation. Till then we can at best hope to stage a holding action against TB and other infections that plague the poor countries of the world.

It is inconceivable to visualize even a distant future in which man and medicine have banished all infections. There is a remarkable ecological balance between man and his microscopic fellow creatures. It is impossible to destroy all the pathogenic organisms with powerful antibiotics, for nature breeds resistant strains that continue to cause disease. Resistant pneumococci, staphylococcus, resistant gram-negative organisms particularly those belonging to the enterobacter species pose grave dangers today in many parts of the world. The indiscriminate use of antibiotics disrupts the ecological balance between man and micro-organisms and is perilous to the safety of man.

In fact it is more than likely that the future world will witness new diseases and new infections. New disease could result from changes in social and environmental conditions. Micro-organisms and in particular viruses can mutate for known and unknown reasons. They can then produce new infections and diseases never encountered earlier in the history of man. The HIV is an example of a virus, which has probably mutated several times before it struck our contemporary world.

Health problems in the future world will be accentuated by the anticipated population explosion in the poor countries. A recent UN report projected that the world population could reach 9.4 billion by 2050. A statistical study identifies 28 countries (20 of them in Africa) where the fertility rate increased during the past decade. Malthus' gloomy forecast embodied in 'An Essay on the Principle Population as it Affects the Future Improvement of the Society' may still at least in part come true. Feeding the world's masses even with continuing advances in the science of agriculture may prove to be a problem, which may be insoluble in times of war and natural disasters. Just as dangerous will be the uncontrolled consumption of non-renewable resources, the irreversible destruction of habitats and species, the pollution of the air, rivers and seas, and many other dangers of an exploding human population.

Global warming is another phenomenon which if unchecked could lead in the near future to catastrophic events on our planet—events that may well directly or indirectly influence the cause or spread of disease, as also tax medical resources to breaking point, particularly in the poor developing countries of the world. The average global air temperature near the earth's surface increased by 0.74±0.18°C in the year ending 2005. Climate model projections indicate that the global surface temperature will likely rise a further 1.1 to 4°C during the twenty-first century. Most of the observed increase in globally averaged temperature since the mid-twentieth century is due to the observed increase in man-made greenhouse gas concentrations (in particular carbon emissions) via an increased greenhouse effect. Increased global temperature is expected in the future to cause sea levels to rise causing an inundation and perhaps obliteration of some of the islands and coastal areas in our world. There could also be an increase in the intensity of extreme weather events, significant changes in the amount and pattern of precipitation, leading to an increase in the expanse of tropical areas and an increase in its degree of deforestation. Global warming could reduce agricultural yields, induce glacial melting and species extinction. Natural disasters in the form of floods, famines, could plague the earth.

Climatic changes in conjunction with natural disasters could in the future markedly increase the burden of diseases all over the world, particularly in poor countries which remarkably enough, contribute the least to the emission of greenhouse gases and greenhouse effect. Global warming is expected to increase the potential geographic range and virulence of tropical disease. Climate changes could also cause a major increase in insect-borne disease, such as malaria throughout Europe, North America and North Asia.

Limiting industrial emission of greenhouse gases is the only solution to reduce and perhaps arrest global warming. This would involve adopting alternate energy sources in order to reduce carbon emissions. All countries of the world must come together and jointly fight a menace that can endanger many aspects of our future world.

The Future World

Future medicine will reflect the future world. Quantum science of the twentieth century gave birth to the biomolecular and computer age, ushering in revolutions that have changed the world and will continue to do so in an exponential manner. We have given a brief glimpse of the future potential of the biomolecular and biotechnical revolutions. The computer revolution has also strongly influenced both man and medicine and will increasingly do so in the years to come. It is the computer, which has spawned information technology, introduced the world to the Internet, abolished our age-old concept of time and space and promises in the future to knit the world in a tighter, closer embrace.

Michio Kaku, an internationally known theoretical physicist and the Henry Sernat professor at The City University of New York, is of the opinion that the Quantum theory will in the near future give us nanotechnology—the ability to make machines the size of atoms, thereby ushering another industrial revolution. Professor Kaku forecasts the possibility of a tiny computer, the size of atoms, inserted into our blood stream, giving us continuous data on our health and at the same time correcting any deviations from health that may arise within us. He contends that by 2020 according to Moore's law computer chips will cost next to nothing—perhaps less than a scrap of paper. All appliances will be computerized. Prototypes already exist of a) the Internet watch—one talks to it and it talks back assessing the whole database of the Internet; b) the intelligent tie-clasp which has the combined power of a laptop and the cell phone; c) the Geo-Positioning Earring which will access the Geo-Positioning Satellites in orbit and give the wearer his or her location within 20 feet; d) smart spectacles which will video image a medical conference in the wearers' eye-glasses; e) smart clothes and toilet —the clothes will monitor the wearer's health and in case of a heart attack will automatically call the ambulance to the exact location. Professor Kaku mentions that the Japanese are already marketing a smart toilet, which automatically analyzes one's body fluids.

The dream of scientists is to create true artificial intelligence. Is a computer brain possible? Raymond Ruszweil, author of *Age of Spiritual Machines*, contends that scientists have already replicated input output characteristics of clusters of hundreds of neurones. Is there a possibility of scaling up from hundreds of neurones to billions of neurones that the human brain contains, and of computing further than 500 trillion bytes per second as our human brain does? Even if this becomes possible in the distant future there are certain human qualities which a machine however intelligent can never possess—for these are qualities which are not directly related or linked to intelligence. How can a machine ever possess imagination, experience, wisdom, intuition and above all how can it blossom into a spirituality that was the essence of great prophets such as Zoroaster, Buddha, Mahavir, Christ, or on a lesser plane of great human beings such as Hippocrates, Charaka, Susruta, or Martin Luther King, Mahatma Gandhi, Mother Theresa?

Many an eminent scientist believes that 'consciousness' and 'intelligence' are not the same. Sir John Eccles, a famous scientist and a Nobel laureate in his Gifford lectures writes that 'consciousness' is distinct from 'thinking' or 'intelligence'. 'The unity of conscious experience is provided by the self-conscious mind and not by the neuronal machinery of the liaison areas of the cerebral hemispheres.' And what is the self-conscious mind? How has it come about? This indeed is the mystery of life, a mystery that may well be beyond the grasp of future science. Eccles considers the self-conscious mind as a self-subsistent entity which integrates the multifarious activities of the neuronal machinery to give the unity of conscious existence from moment to moment.

Ethical Questions

Future medicine will pose grave moral and ethical questions. The pace of development in the science of genetics in relation to reproduction and procreation has far outstripped the pace at which ethical questions are being resolved. Bioethics is an uncharted sea and we need to map and chart this sea if humanity is not to be wrecked on its shoals and reefs. It is not within the scope of this essay to discuss at length the numerous ethical and moral issues raised by medical science now and in the future. I shall confine myself to a brief discussion of the ethical quandary that can result from manipulation of the human genome, and from advances in genetic advancement and genetic engineering.

The future will need to ensure the freedom of scientific research and yet safeguard the respect for fundamental human rights; it will need to strike a balance between science and humanity for the benefit of man and medicine. The General Conference of UNESCO in November 1997 discussed these issues and adopted the 'Declaration on the Human Genome and Human Rights'. The Declaration considered the explosion in genetic engineering techniques, their application in medicine and the fundamental rights of man to exercise choice. The Declaration further states that freedom of research is part of freedom of thought and is necessary for the progress of knowledge. It maintains that the application of research in genetics, biology and medicine, concerning the human genome must be directed to the relief of suffering and improving the health of individuals and of humankind. Within three years of this declaration, the human genome was unravelled and deciphered. The fallout of this landmark discovery in medicine has sent reverberations through the scientific world.

Many scientists are unhappy with the UNESCO declaration of 1997. It is impossible to ban or curb freedom of thought or of research that goes with the freedom of thought. They feel that freedom to research should not be confined merely to the relief of human suffering; the freedom should be unbridled and allow man to meet the challenges that could result from manipulation of the human embryo through genetic enhancement and genetic engineering.

The evolutionary history of man stretches back millions and millions of years. Man has not ceased to evolve—he will continue to do so, perhaps indefinitely, through the corridors of time, unless he destroys himself or is destroyed during this passage. However, his evolution through genetic drift or Darwinian natural selection to a point where he is significantly different from his present state or 'being' may take many many more million years. The science of genetics can conceivably achieve the further evolution of man in perhaps a few hundred or thousand years. The debate is whether science should be given the unfettered freedom to pursue this dream. It is the old Baconian vision that is being revived, the dream to master nature 'for the relief of man's estate' and usher in a different but 'brave new world' envisioned by Aldous Huxley far back in 1936. This world would liberate man from moral, emotional, physical constraints and go many steps further to even liberate him from his present biological state, helping him evolve into a 'super-being'. To many, a world such as this has many attractive facets; for it promises good health, longevity, freedom from anxiety and from moral constraints, sex without love and restraint. Huxley, however, realized that these 'desires' could only be attained by forgoing the higher attributes that man is endowed with—a Faustian exchange, a barter of the soul which is so subtle that those who make this choice will neither see or realize it.

Will the future see this dream come true, or will the dream turn into a nightmare? Will the future be close to heaven or will it be a living hell?

Those unconnected with science would perhaps disbelieve what I have written. How could the science of genetics change man to a different species unrecognizable to us today? They would consider this possibility a figment of a vivid imagination, science fiction stretched to absurdity. But this is not true. Let me quote a few news items from early 2001 to show those uninitiated in science how pressing and relevant the problem is.

'Scientists have created the first genetically modified monkey, an advance that could lead to customized primates for medical research and that brings the possibility of genetic manipulation closer than ever to humans.'

—*Washington Post*, 12 January, 2001

'Among the NIH funded studies, is one in California in which human foetal tissues have been transplanted into mice to create rodents with humanised immune systems.'

—*Washington Post*, 26 January, 2001

'Late last year, genetic engineering watchdog groups warned that the European Union had granted a patent in December 1999 to an Australian company for a process that would allow the creation of chimerical creatures—human / animal hybrids –

The patent specifically covers the possible creation of embryos containing cells from humans and mice, sheep, pigs, cattle, goats or fish'.

—*National Catholic Register*, 28 January, 2001.

These are animal experiments in genetic engineering; they may well be a precursor to similar experiments on humans. We are not dealing with absurd science fiction. We are dealing with a scenario well within the realm of possibility. There are many opponents who feel that unbridled freedom to scientific research on genetic enhancement and genetic engineering could prove a disaster to the human race. It would be unethical and immoral to allow the application of scientific research on the human genome to prevail over respect for human rights and dignity. In my opinion, it would be dangerous to trespass into the future and use the power of science so that only good genes prevail and that the 'not so good genes' are eliminated. If man and medicine were to counter nature and the process of natural selection, would the world have seen Homer, Toulouse-Lautrec, Helen Keller or Stephen Hawking? To consider every genetic defect in the human genome as a tragedy that needs to be extinguished at its very origin violates dignity and rights. Genetic engineering to cure diseases such as cystic fibrosis or defects such as muscular dystrophy is welcome and is to be encouraged. But to trespass into the future and use the science of genetics to alter our DNA and genome radically, with a view to encode our vanities, change our attributes or what is even more sinister, quickly evolve into new life forms, into a new super-race is wrong and fraught with danger. We must tread carefully if our world in the future is not to become a stage for a true-to-life Greek tragedy.

We have evolved over well-nigh countless years into a distinct species. We encode within our genomic history and development not just increasing intelligence but other higher attributes—consciousness i.e. self-awareness, love, compassion, charity, justice—attributes peculiar to our species. We will continue to change and evolve, for evolution is a 'marker' of all life. If we go by what has already transpired and tread the same evolutionary path, we should evolve perhaps into even better human beings with a greater abundance of the higher attributes that distinguish us from other species in this world.

If we however whittle down the evolutionary path dictated by the science of genetics, condensing our evolution to a few hundred or a few thousand years we may cease to be human. We may just be dehumanized artefacts. Artefacts that are perhaps, stronger, bigger, more intelligent, more beautiful and equipped for even further genetic enhancements. Yet artefacts may be devoid of any worthy values and therefore in many ways truly subhuman and fit for the jungle.

Cloning of humans is another debatable issue. It has been banned by governments and official bodies but it can always be accomplished clandestinely. The moral philosophy that most scientists today consider worth following is that of Immanuel Kant, the moralist and philosopher of the nineteenth century. Kant considered each human being as an individual and as an end but not as a means to an end. Under this moral precept, cloning stands as unethical and undesirable. There is always the possibility of science being reduced to depravity and made to clone Frankensteins. Even otherwise, humans clones will be means to an end, they will not be valued as individuals in their own right but as copies of others we respected or loved. Yet there are a number of scientists with liberal views who believe that there should never be a padlock on scientific research, never a restraint on the freedom of inquiry. They view the ban on cloning as a 'triumph of superstition, government coercion, self-righteousness and fear over good sense, health, family values and confidence in the future'. They further contend that if humans have a right to reproduce, society has no right to limit the means. They evidently believe that the means justifies the end, though with regard to human cloning, most people contend that both the means and the end are reprehensible. Leon A. Katz writing in the book *The Future is Now* (Editors William Kristel and Eric Cohen) gives cogent arguments against human cloning. He maintains that an attempt to clone a human being is an unethical experiment on the human child-to-be. This is because animal experiments have shown that only two to three per cent of cloning attempts have succeeded, and of the successful animal clones many are diseased or deformed. Therefore attempts to produce human clones carry unacceptable massive risks of producing deformed healthy children. What would one do with such children—destroy them, discard them? Even if technology improves to a point where human cloning is successful, the clone may experience serious problems with regard to his or her identity and individuality. A further argument is that human cloning would transform the act of 'begetting' children into 'making' children, of procreation into manufacture. Man himself could then become one of the so many other 'man-made things'. Finally Katz very correctly emphasizes that procreation converted to manufacture would with almost certainty allow the making of cloned babies a profitable commercial proposition. We would then enter into an era where the sale of cloned babies having requisite characteristics would be on par with the sale of other commodities!!

At best, human cloning is the most extreme form of narcissism—a narcissism, which is both authoritarian and despotic, for it is designed to 'make' a child in one's own image and impose a future according to one's own will. At worst human cloning may populate our own world with Frankensteins—monsters that could destroy our planet. It is more likely for those such as Hitler, Mussolini or Stalin to desire their own clones than for an Einstein, Newton or a Kepler to do so. Let me dwell just for one moment on an even more sickening scenario. Scientists have cloned headless mice and there are prominent scientists who see the possibility of ultimately creating headless human clones for the purpose of organ harvesting. For if you create a headless clone of just your body you have created a source of replacement organs that could keep you going indefinitely. A nightmare that makes one shudder to the core!

There are therefore truly cogent reasons to ban cloning, though how successful such a ban would be is impossible to foretell. There should be no exceptions to this ban. We are not on the proverbial slippery slope, we stand on the peak of a very steep high cliff—we need to step back.

The moral and ethical questions raised in this discussion need to be answered now, for the future is now. Do we have the moral right, the wisdom, the ethical consent to prefabricate and design our descendants? It is already late; very soon the choice will not be in our hands. Even if we do make a choice, is it possible to enforce it? Could we stop a new genetically engineered evolution of humankind, even if we wanted to?

The future of man and medicine rests with man. He should not be blinded by the dazzling light of science, nor bewitched by its power and beauty so as to be servile to it. He should channelize it for the benefit of mankind, subjecting it to ethical and moral constraints. If he does so, man and medicine in the distant future may usher in *a truly brave new world*—not the brave new world envisioned by Aldous Huxley. If he fails to do so, mankind will once again be plunged into 'a new Dark Age made more sinister and perhaps more protracted by the lights of perverted science'.